The ECT Handbook

Second Edition

The ECT Handbook

Second Edition

The Third Report of the
Royal College of Psychiatrists'
Special Committee on ECT

Edited by
Allan I. F. Scott

Council Report CR128
Approved by Council: January 2004
Due for review: 2009

Royal College of Psychiatrists

The Royal College of Psychiatrists,
17 Belgrave Square, London SW1X 8PG
http://www.rcpsych.ac.uk

British Library Cataloguing-in-Publication Data
A catalogue record for this book is available from the British Library.
ISBN 1-904671-22-5

Distributed in North America by Balogh International Inc.

Printed in Great Britain by Bell & Bain Limited, Glasgow.

Contents

Part II. Psychotropic drug treatment and ECT

Part III. The administration of ECT

Part IV. The law and consent

Appendices

Figures

Contributors

Dr **Ian Anderson**, Senior Lecturer in Psychiatry, Neuroscience and Psychiatry Unit, University of Manchester

Dr **Richard Barnes**, Consultant in Old Age Psychiatry, Mossley Hill Hospital, Liverpool

Professor **Susan M. Benbow**, Professor of Mental Health and Ageing, University of Wolverhampton, and Consultant Old Age Psychiatrist, Wolverhampton City Primary Care Trust

Dr **C. John Bowley**, Consultant Anaesthetist, City Hospital and Queen's Medical Centre, Nottingham

Mrs **Linda Cullen**, Project Nurse, Scottish ECT Audit Network, Royal Edinburgh Hospital

Dr **Richard Duffett**, Consultant Psychiatrist, Goodmayes Hospital, Essex

Dr **Jim A. T. Dyer**, OBE, Former Director, Mental Welfare Commission for Scotland

Dr **Andrew Easton**, Consultant Psychiatrist, Newsam Centre, Seacroft Hospital, Leeds

Dr **Christopher F. Fear**, Consultant Psychiatrist, Wotton Lawn Hospital, Gloucester

Dr **Grace M. Fergusson**, Consultant Psychiatrist, Argyll and Bute Hospital, Lochgilphead

Professor **I. Nicol Ferrier**, Professor of Psychiatry, School of Neurology, Neurobiology and Psychiatry, University of Newcastle, Newcastle upon Tyne

Dr **Chris P. Freeman**, Consultant Psychotherapist, Royal Edinburgh Hospital

Dr Ennapadam S. Krishnamoorthy, Specialist Registrar in Neurology, University Department of Clinical Neurology, Institute of Neurology, London

Dr Heinrich C. Lamprecht, Specialist Registrar in Old Age Psychiatry, Newcastle General Hospital, Newcastle upon Tyne

Dr Stephen M. Lawrie, Senior Clinical Research Fellow, Division of Psychiatry, University of Edinburgh

Professor Keith Matthews, Professor of Psychiatry and Chair, Special Committee on ECT, Division of Pathology and Neuroscience, University of Dundee, Ninewells Hospital and Medical School

Professor Roy J. McClelland, Professor of Mental Health, Queen's University, Belfast

Dr Andrew M. McIntosh, Clinical Research Fellow, Division of Psychiatry, University of Edinburgh

Dr Bruce Moore, Consultant Psychiatrist, Halton General Hospital, Runcorn

Dr Walter J. Muir, Reader in the Psychiatry of Learning Disability, Division of Psychiatry, University of Edinburgh

Professor Ian C. Reid, Professor of Psychiatry, Institute of Medical Sciences, University of Aberdeen

Dr Allan I. F. Scott, Consultant Psychiatrist, Royal Edinburgh Hospital

Dr Martin Stevens, Consultant Psychiatrist, Ipswich Hospital

Dr Alan G. Swann, Consultant Psychiatrist in Old Age Psychiatry, Newcastle General Hospital, Newcastle upon Tyne

Professor Michael R. Trimble, Professor of Behavioural Neurology, Institute of Neurology, Queen Square, London

Dr Heather A. C. Walker, Consultant Anaesthetist, North Manchester General Hospital

Dr Andrew M. Whitehouse, Consultant Psychiatrist, University Hospital, Nottingham

Introduction

This edition of *The ECT Handbook* will be published later than was anticipated when the first edition was written in 1994. In the year 2000, the Secretary of State for Health commissioned two systematic reviews of ECT, one on its efficacy and safety and the other on the attitudes of patients towards it. Subsequently and separately, the National Institute for Clinical Excellence (NICE) commissioned a Health Technology Appraisal of ECT for depressive illness, schizophrenia, catatonia and mania. These findings became available only during 2003 (see Chapter 1). In the same year, the Royal College of Psychiatrists announced its plan for the College Research Unit to establish an ECT Accreditation Service that would inspect ECT clinics.

The present edition has been able to take account of these developments, and should assist prescribers and practitioners of ECT in the review of their practice in the light of these findings and recommendations. A particular challenge from the NICE guidance is that we strive to reduce further the possibility that patients suffer cognitive adverse effects attributable to ECT.

The Special Committee wishes to promote the use of a unilateral electrode placement in non-urgent treatments (see Chapters 1, 2 and 15), and recommends further refinements to stimulus dosing (see Chapters 2 and 16). The Committee also recommends that monitoring by electroencephalogram be available in all ECT clinics from 1 January 2006 (see Chapter 17).

The formal recommendations and good practice points from the Special Committee are given in Chapters 1–20. The Appendices do not contain such formal recommendations, but are provided as resources for ECT practitioners.

This edition does not include a College factsheet for patients and carers. The College has decided, in line with the NICE guidance, that the production of such a leaflet should be undertaken separately, as a public information exercise, and involve representatives of users, carers, other professional organisations and the voluntary sector.

The College's Special Committee on ECT started to provide regular training courses in the practice of ECT in 1992; these will continue and the content will evolve to match those set out in this Handbook. In 2002, the Committee first organised a national forum for more experienced staff, 'The Practitioners' Day', and such events will continue to be held.

My thanks go to all those who have helped in the production of these guidelines. Special thanks must go to Ms Alex Celini, who supported the work of the Committee, and to Ms Fiona Morrison, who took on a heavy commitment in the production and revision of the manuscripts.

Dr Allan I. F. Scott
Special Committee on ECT
January 2005

Part I
Clinical guidelines

CHAPTER 1

The place of ECT in contemporary psychiatric practice

The Consensus Group Affiliated to the Special Committee*

While this second edition of the *ECT Handbook* was in production, the National Institute for Clinical Excellence (NICE) was commissioned to undertake a Health Technology Appraisial of ECT in the treatment of depressive illness, mania, schizophrenia and catatonia. The Royal College of Psychiatrists was consulted as part of the appraisal process and in particular was asked to produce a position statement about the place of ECT in contemporary psychiatric practice. The Special Committee on ECT consulted psychiatrists with expertise in the application of ECT, encompassing both academic and clinical experience. This included the outcome of consultation with consultant psychiatrists with responsibility for ECT clinics in trusts around the UK who attended the ECT Practitioners' Day at the King's Fund under the auspices of the College on 11 October 2002. This led to the formation of the Consensus Group, who later wrote this position statement. The Group consisted of psychiatrists from the Special Committee, other contributors to the present edition and delegates at the Practitioner's Day (see note below). The findings of two important systematic reviews sponsored by the Department of Health were presented and discussed on the day. These were the review of the efficacy and safety of ECT carried out by the UK ECT Review Group (2003) and that of consumers' perspectives carried out by the Service User Research Enterprise (Rose *et al*, 2003). These systematic reviews left several important clinical questions unanswered. It was therefore necessary to consider evidence apart from randomised controlled trials, tempered by the Group's expert judgement based on clinical experience. The Consensus Group produced the position

*The members of the Consensus Group were Dr Ian Anderson, Dr Richard Barnes, Professor Susan Benbow, Dr Richard Duffett, Dr Andrew Easton, Dr Chris Fear, Dr Grace Fergusson, Professor Nicol Ferrier, Dr Chris Freeman, Dr Heinrich Lamprecht, Professor Keith Matthews, Dr Bruce Moore, Dr Allan Scott, Dr Martin Stevens, Dr Alan Swann and Dr Andrew Whitehouse.

statement on contemporary indications for the use of ECT, which was presented to NICE in October 2002. The main recommendations presented in that statement are considered below, along with the guidance produced by NICE and the Consensus Group's response to that guidance.

Recommendations of the Consensus Group's position statement

Major depressive episode/disorder

Electroconvulsive therapy may be the treatment of choice for severe depressive illness when there is an urgent need for treatment, for example when the depressive illness is associated with:

- attempted suicide
- strong suicidal ideas or plans
- life-threatening illness because of the patient's refusal of food or fluids.

Electroconvulsive therapy may be considered for the treatment of severe depressive illness associated with:

- stupor
- marked psychomotor retardation
- depressive delusions or hallucinations.

In the absence of the above, ECT may be considered as a second- or third-line treatment of a depressive illness that has not adequately responded to antidepressant drug treatment and where social recovery has not been achieved (e.g. an inability to return to work). Initial treatment failure may be defined as a lack of recovery after a course of an antidepressant drug given at a proven effective dose for at least 6 weeks (with the exception of elderly sufferers, who may take longer to respond to antidepressant drug treatment). A switch to an antidepressant drug with a different mode of action is the preferred second-line treatment. If the depressive illness persists, several options are available, namely, adding an augmenting agent, such as lithium carbonate or tri-iodothyronine, switching to a monoamine oxidase inhibitor for patients with atypical major depression, adding either cognitive therapy or another form of psychotherapy, or switching to ECT.

Patient choice is important. Some sufferers who have previously had a depressive illness may choose ECT because of their experience of medical treatment that was ineffective or intolerable, or previous experience of recovery with ECT.

Mania

The treatment of choice for mania is a mood-stabilising drug plus an antipsychotic drug. ECT may be considered for severe mania associated with:

- life-threatening physical exhaustion
- treatment resistance (i.e. mania that has not responded to the treatment of choice).

Patient choice and a previous experience of ineffective or intolerable medical treatment, or previous recovery with ECT, are again relevant.

Acute schizophrenia

The treatment of choice for acute schizophrenia is antipsychotic drug treatment. ECT may be considered as a fourth-line option, that is, for patients with schizophrenia for whom clozapine has already proven ineffective or intolerable.

Catatonia

Catatonia is a syndrome that may complicate several psychiatric and medical conditions. The treatment of choice is a benzodiazepine drug; most experience is with lorazepam. ECT may be indicated when treatment with lorazepam has been ineffective.

NICE guidance

In May 2003 NICE published its guidance on ECT for depressive illness, schizophrenia, catatonia and mania (NICE, 2003a). This was simultaneously endorsed by NHS Quality Improvement Scotland. The guidance about the indications for ECT in these conditions included the following statements:

'ECT is used only to achieve rapid and short-term improvement of severe symptoms after an adequate trial of other treatment options has proven ineffective and/or when the condition is considered to be potentially life-threatening, in individuals with:

- severe depressive illness
- catatonia
- a prolonged or severe manic episode.'

'The current state of the evidence does not allow the general use of ECT in the management of schizophrenia to be recommended.'

'As the longer-term benefits and risks of ECT have not been clearly established, it is not recommended as a maintenance therapy in depressive illness.'

'The decision as to whether ECT is clinically indicated should be based on a documented assessment of the risks and potential benefits to the individual, including: the risks associated with the anaesthetic, contemporaneous co-morbidities, anticipated adverse events, particularly cognitive impairment, and the risks of not having treatment.'

'The risks associated with ECT may be enhanced during pregnancy, in older people and in children and young people, and therefore clinicians should exercise particular caution when considering ECT in these groups.'

A media briefing released at the same time (NICE, 2003*b*) included the following statement:

'The [Appraisal] Committee took special note of the evidence from observations of users' experiences relating to the adverse effects of ECT. In particular, cognitive impairment following ECT was discussed in detail. It was apparent that cognitive impairment often out-weighed their perception of any benefit from ECT treatment. These factors featured significantly in the Committee's decision to restrict the use of ECT to situations in which all other alternatives had been exhausted or where the nature of the mental illness was considered to be "life-threatening".'

Response of the Consensus Group to the guidance

The guidance and the indications suggested in the Consensus Group's position statement were in the main consistent regarding the contemporary indications for ECT in mania, acute schizophrenia and catatonia. They were not consistent about the place of ECT in major depression, the illness for which the treatment is most commonly prescribed. The Consensus Group therefore reconvened to produce the following response, which it is hoped will help practitioners to accommodate the NICE guidance in their clinical practice.

Observations on the NICE guidance on the indications for ECT in major depression

Divergence from the NICE guidance would occur if a practitioner were considering the prescription of ECT for depressive illness that was not life-threatening or severe, that was not demonstrably resistant to alternative treatments, or as continuation or maintenance treatment. In these cases the Consensus Group would make the following observations:

- Health professionals are expected to take NICE guidance fully into account when exercising their clinical judgement. NICE guidance does not, however, override the individual responsibility of health professionals to make decisions appropriate to the circumstances of the individual patient, in consultation with the patient and/or guardian or carer.

- The NICE guidance on ECT does not have any legal jurisdiction over clinical practice, and its legal significance could be established only if it were cited in a court case.

- A documented assessment of the potential risks and benefits of treatment to which valid consent has been obtained would be essential to support any variance from the NICE guidance. The Royal College of Psychiatrists' Special Committee on ECT has already recommended the safeguard of obtaining a second opinion from an independent psychiatrist when the indication is potentially controversial. This may be prudent too were any variance from the NICE guidance being considered. The patient may also be able to express a clear view about the perceived severity of the illness and the role of ECT in its treatment; this should be documented.

- The thrust of the NICE guidance is that the therapeutic benefits of ECT may be outweighed by the distress caused when patients realise they have suffered lengthy or permanent retrograde amnesia. Patients who have never before been treated with ECT will be less able to consider the trade-off between the immediate benefit and this longer-term risk. Practitioners ought therefore to exercise particular circumspection in the use of ECT at variance with the NICE guidance in patients with depression who have never before been treated with ECT. It would be prudent to be particularly careful to discuss the topic of retrograde amnesia, particularly for personal memories, and to document this discussion.

- The cognitive adverse effects of ECT can be substantially reduced by the use of a unilateral electrode placement and, to a lesser extent, by the avoidance of substantially supra-threshold electrical doses. This strategy is strongly recommended as the initial treatment in any prescription beyond the NICE guidance. It would in any case be good practice in the treatment of illnesses that are not life-threatening or severe.

- Practitioners may also have to consider ECT beyond the NICE guidance when it is requested by a patient. The guidance makes reference to the view that the wishes of the patient must be of paramount importance. Further clarification from NICE suggests that this is not meant to support consumerism among patients, but to support the view that valid and informed consent is necessary for the appropriate prescription for ECT. The same circumspection and documented risk–benefit analysis would be required here, as in other indications.

Acknowledgements

We thank Ms Alex Celini & Ms Fiona Morrison for their help in collating the work of the Group and in the production of the manuscript.

References

NICE (2003a) *Guidance on the Use of Electroconvulsive Therapy.* Technology Appraisal 59. London: NICE. Available at http://www.nice.org.uk/pdf/59ectfullguidance.pdf

NICE (2003b) Media briefing. Available at http://www.nice.org.uk/pdf/59ectmediabriefing.pdf.

Rose, D., Wykes, T., Leese, M., *et al* (2003) Patients' perspectives on electro-convulsive therapy: a systematic review. *British Medical Journal*, **326**, 1363–1365.

UK ECT Review Group (2003) Efficacy and safety of electro-convulsive therapy in depressive disorders: a systematic review and meta-analysis. *Lancet*, **361**, 799–808.

CHAPTER 2

The use of ECT in depressive illness

Heinrich C. Lamprecht, I. Nicol Ferrier and Alan G. Swann

Since the publication of the previous edition of *The ECT Handbook* in 1995, the use of ECT has not become less controversial. The arrival of several new antidepressants and atypical antipsychotics has fuelled the debate even further. We aim in this chapter to give objective evidence for the efficacy of ECT and practical guidelines for its use in depression.

Efficacy of ECT in depression

Data for the efficacy of ECT in depression are taken from the systematic review of its efficacy and safety sponsored by the Department of Health (UK ECT Review Group, 2003). The results on efficacy were based on randomised control trials (RCTs) identified in an extensive search. Search results were independently checked by two reviewers. Studies that satisfied the inclusion criteria were distributed to paired members of the review team for data extraction and any disagreements were resolved by group discussion. All the identified trials were assessed according to methodological aspects of trial design that have been shown to affect the validity of results. Where appropriate, data from individual trials were summarised by meta-analyses.

ECT versus 'sham' ECT

There is a substantial body of evidence to support the efficacy of ECT. Six RCTs comparing ECT with 'sham' ECT in the short-term treatment of depression have presented data on a total of 256 patients (Wilson *et al*, 1963; Lambourn & Gill, 1978; Freeman *et al*, 1978; Johnstone *et al*, 1980; West, 1981; Gregory *et al*, 1985). These were mainly in-patients under the age of 70 with heterogeneous diagnoses of depression. The depression ratings at the end of treatment showed the standardised effect size (SES) between real and simulated ECT to be -0.91 (95% CI $= -1.27$ to -0.54), indicating a mean difference in the Hamilton Rating Scale for Depression (HRSD) of 9.67 (95% CI $= 5.72$ to 13.53) in favour of ECT.

ECT versus pharmacotherapy

There were 18 RCTs with 1144 patients in total comparing ECT with drug therapy in the short-term treatment of depression. Of these, 13 had enough data to contribute to a pooled analysis. The SES of these trials is –0.80 (95% CI= –1.29 to –0.29). This translates to a mean difference of 5.2 (95% CI = 1.37 to 8.87) on the HRSD in favour of ECT, indicating that ECT is more effective than drug therapy in the treatment of depression. None of these trials compared ECT with newer anti-depressant medications such as the selective serotonin reuptake inhibitors (SSRIs), mirtazepine or venlafaxine.

Bilateral versus unilateral ECT

The data from 21 studies could be used to calculate an SES of bilateral versus unilateral application of ECT. Various electrode placements were used in both bilateral and unilateral ECT. In only eight of these was a duration of treatment described. There was an SES of –0.32 (95% CI= –0.46 to –0.20) in favour of bilateral ECT.

It is impossible to do a meta-analysis on the data evaluating cognitive function in these trials, as different cognitive tests were used. Some studies concentrated more on anterograde than on retrograde memory and some vice versa. In those reporting on overall cognitive function, bilateral ECT caused statistically greater impairment on some tests of cognitive function either in the first week (Heshe *et al*, 1978) or the second week (Sackeim *et al*, 2000*b*). There were, however, no statistical differences at 2 months (Sackeim *et al*, 1993) or at 3 months (Heshe *et al*, 1978). Two studies reported on long-term outcome. Weiner *et al* (1986) found no difference in anterograde memory but long-term personal memory was more impaired in the group who received bilateral ECT. Bidder *et al* (1970) found no differences in verbal memory at 1 year.

Frequency of ECT

In clinical practice ECT is sometimes administered initially three times a week to patients with more severe depression, although there is no objective evidence for this practice. Six trials, involving a total of 210 patients, were available. Four compared twice-weekly with thrice-weekly ECT (Kellner *et al*, 1992; Lerer *et al*, 1995; Janakiramaiah *et al*, 1998*a*; Vieweg & Shawcross, 1998) and two compared once-weekly with thrice-weekly ECT (Gangadhar *et al*, 1993; Shapira *et al*, 1998). Analysing them separately and together showed no difference in favour of ECT given three times a week: the SES of twice versus three times a week was –0.30 (95% CI = –0.76 to 0.20) and the SES of once versus three times a week was 0.83 (95% CI = –0.39 to 1.89). When analysed together, the mean change in HRSD score was not statistically significant, 0.40 (95% CI = –5.26 to 6.30).

Four of these trials reported on cognitive function (Kellner *et al*, 1992; Lerer *et al*, 1995; Shapira *et al*, 1998; Vieweg & Shawcross, 1998) but a meta-analysis to compare the effect on cognitive function of ECT given two versus three times a week was not possible, due to different measures used.

Dose of electrical stimulus

Trials were divided into higher- and lower-dose stimulation. There were seven trials, involving a total of 342 patients. Six of these (317 patients) reported enough data to contribute to a pooled analyses (Robin & de Tissera, 1982; Sackeim *et al*, 1993, 2000*a*; McCall *et al*, 1995, 2000; Janakiramaiah *et al*, 1998*b*). There was a mean difference in the HRSD score of 5.24 (95% CI = 2.94 to 7.75) in favour of the higher-dose group.

Number of ECT sessions/extra sessions of ECT

There is no evidence to indicate what number of sessions of ECT gains the best response. Neither is there any evidence to support the practice of giving two extra ECT sessions after the patient is considered to be well enough to discontinue ECT.

The place of ECT in the treatment of depression

There has been a general decline in the use of ECT which is much steeper in general adult psychiatry compared with old age psychiatry (Eranti & McLoughlin, 2003). The reasons for the more marked reduction in the younger patients may be:

• the use of evidence-based medicine resulting in a narrowing of the group of illnesses for which ECT is claimed to be effective
• the advent of newer antidepressants
• the use of atypical antipsychotics in depressive psychoses.

If practitioners have less personal experience of the selection of patients for ECT and of its efficacy, then this too may contribute to the decline in usage. None the less, ECT still has a place in the treatment of depression, as discussed below.

The use of ECT in the emergency treatment of depression

As an emergency treatment, ECT is mainly used for patients with a severe depressive episode and severe psychomotor retardation with associated problems of eating and drinking or physical deterioration. It is also used in patients with depression who are actively suicidal. The use of ECT as a primary intervention is based on its efficacy (as proven above) and speed of working. How rapid this is differs between patients, but substantial and sustained improvements have been demonstrated after one to three treatments (Rodger *et al*, 1994), with nearly maximum improvements in some patients after two weeks of ECT three times per week (Post *et al*, 1987). Although it has been suggested that it is effective only in severe depressive psychosis or psychomotor retardation (Buchan *et al*, 1992), more recent evidence suggests an early improvement in all subtypes of depression (Sobin *et al*, 1996) and it should therefore be considered as a possible first-line treatment in all emergencies (Porter & Ferrier, 1999).

In emergencies bilateral ECT should be administered, as it is more effective than unilateral ECT; it also works faster, given an equivalent electrical dose, and high-dose bilateral ECT works faster than low-dose bilateral ECT (Sackeim *et al*, 1993). As discussed above, there is no evidence that administering ECT three times a week improves the final outcome, but there is some evidence that the response is more rapid (Shapira *et al*, 1998). If there are significant cognitive side-effects and a decision is made to switch to unilateral ECT, the 'Lancaster' unilateral electrode placement should not be used, as it does not achieve sufficiently wide separation of the electrodes. The d'Elia position should be used (see Chapter 16). Higher-dose unilateral ECT is more effective than lower-dose unilateral ECT. 'High dose' was defined as 2.5 times the seizure threshold in a double-blind controlled trial by Sackeim *et al* (1993). Higher dosage yet may make unilateral ECT more efficacious, but carries the risk of increased cognitive impairment.

Coexisting physical illnesses are more common in emergencies. It is generally safe to treat such patients with ECT because of the advances in the practice of ECT and because there are no absolute contra-indications for ECT (see Chapter 7).

We therefore recommend bilateral ECT in a dose 50–100% above seizure threshold in dire emergencies, for instance where patients are dehydrated, stuporose or extremely suicidal (Porter & Ferrier, 1999). In less-pressing situations, we concur with the suggestion of Lock (1995) that unilateral ECT in a dose at least 200% above seizure threshold should be used, that is, at least three times the seizure threshold.

The use of ECT in the treatment of depression

It has frequently been reported that ECT is more effective in the treatment of depressed patients with delusions or retardation. Real ECT was no more effective than simulated treatment in patients lacking retardation or delusions (Buchan *et al*, 1992). The opinion has therefore been expressed that ECT should be reserved for depressed patients who have either one or both these features (Lock & McCulloch, 1991; Buchan *et al*, 1992). However, two more recent trials have raised doubts about this perception. Both found that the efficacy of ECT was similar across depressive subtypes. There was no indication that any of the subgroups defined by the presence or absence of psychosis, retardation or agitation displayed a preferential response to ECT (O'Leary et al, 1995; Sobin et al, 1996).

The following factors should influence a decision to use ECT as a first-line treatment in depression:

- the speed and efficacy of ECT
- a patient history of treatment-resistant depression (see below)
- the patient's medication intolerance
- the patient's previous positive response to ECT
- the patient's medical status.

Given ECT's efficacy in depression, it should not be used only as a second-line treatment for depression, nor should it be used only as a last resort.

The use of ECT in treatment-resistant depression

Currently there is no agreed definition of 'treatment-resistant depression'. The Consensus Group (see Chapter 1) suggested that, in the absence of severe symptoms or an urgent need for treatment, treatment resistance should be considered as the failure to respond adequately to two successive courses of monotherapy with pharmacologically different antidepressants given in an adequate dose for sufficient time (Burrows et al, 1994; Fava & Davidson, 1996; Souery et al, 1999; Sackeim, 2001). The proportion of patients who do not respond to either of two anti-depressants is estimated to be 15–20% (Burrows et al, 1994).

Treatment resistance does not rule out a favourable response to ECT. Patients who failed one or more adequate medication trials had a diminished but substantial rate of response to ECT (Prudic et al, 1990, 1996) compared with non-treatment-resistant patients with depression. Even under critical evaluation, ECT can be assumed to be effective in two-thirds to three-quarters of all cases of treatment-resistant depression (Folkerts et al, 1997). There are also trials that have shown no difference in response to ECT in treatment-resistant depression (Kindler et al, 1991; Hussain, 2002). This evidence needs to be considered alongside the patient's risk–benefit ratio for each successive pharmacological treatment (in treatment-resistant depression often multiple, complex and potentially toxic), with the potential benefit weighed against the increasing illness morbidity and likelihood of adverse events or suicide (Nierenberg & Amsterdam, 1990).

The use of ECT in depressive stupor and catatonic depression

In depression, stupor usually follows after a period of increased motor retardation and withdrawal. It is rarely seen nowadays because depressive disorders are diagnosed earlier and are more effectively treated.

Catatonia is a syndrome that may complicate several psychiatric and medical conditions. It is often associated with affective disorder (Abrams & Taylor, 1976; Pataki *et al*, 1992; Bush *et al*, 1996*a*).

According to DSM–IV (American Psychiatric Association, 1994), *catatonic features* are present if the clinical picture is dominated by at least two of the following

- motoric immobility as evidenced by catalepsy (including waxy flexibility) or stupor
- excessive motor activity that is apparently purposeless and not influenced by external stimuli
- extreme negativism or mutism
- peculiarities of voluntary movement, as evidenced by posturing, stereotyped movements, prominent mannerisms or prominent grimacing
- echolalia or echopraxia.

The treatment of choice for catatonia is a benzodiazepine drug. The greatest experience is with lorazepam (Rosebush *et al*, 1990; Ungvari *et al*, 1994; Bush *et al*, 1996*b*), to which most cases respond rapidly. The response to lorazepam on the first day and the duration of catatonia before treatment predicts response (Bush *et al*, 1996*b*). There is no relationship between response to lorazepam and the number of catatonic signs (Abrams & Taylor, 1976). Although benzodiazepines can acutely diminish catatonia, there is no evidence to support their long-term use in catatonia (Swartz *et al*, 2001).

As it is very difficult to distinguish between forms of catatonia, it is important to assess these patients for ECT if catatonia is severe and not relieved by lorazepam within the first few days of treatment (Fricchione, 1989; Pearlman, 1991; Bush *et al*, 1996*b*). The use of neuroleptics is not advised (Taylor, 1990), as they can precipitate catatonic signs (Gellenberg, 1977; Fricchione *et al*, 1983). In a review of 292 cases of 'lethal catatonia', 78.4% of those who received neuroleptics alone died (Mann *et al*, 1986).

In depressive stupor or catatonic stupor we therefore recommend:

- a short-acting benzodiazepine as treatment of first choice
- the referral of these patients for ECT if catatonia is severe and not relieved by a short-acting benzodiazepine within the first few days of treatment.

The use of ECT in treating elderly patients with depression

Electroconvulsive therapy is a highly effective treatment for major depressive disorder in the elderly, perhaps even more so than in younger age groups (Benbow, 1987; Devenand & Kruger, 1994). It is also effective and well tolerated in the 'old-old' (Tew *et al*, 1999). A meta-analyses of outcome studies of use of ECT in the elderly showed that it produced a significant improvement in 83% of cases and remission in 62% (Mulsant *et al*, 1991).

In spite of a higher burden of physical illness, elderly patients with depression are as able as younger, physically healthier patients to complete and benefit from a course of ECT (Tew *et al*, 1999). Tew *et al*'s (1999) results are congruent with those of four previous studies that showed that older physically ill patients respond in a manner similar to younger and physically healthier patients (Alexopoulos *et al*, 1984; Burke *et al*, 1987; Zielinski *et al*, 1993; Rice *et al*, 1994).

Older people tend to have higher seizure thresholds (Wilkinson *et al*, 1993), although age alone predicts only a small proportion of the total variance in seizure threshold. The implications for the practical administration of ECT are covered in Chapters 8 and 16.

Older patients may be more susceptible to confusion after ECT (Burke *et al*, 1987; Mulsant *et al*, 1991; Sackeim, 1992). This should guide decisions regarding the ECT technique employed. Elderly patients and particularly those with pre-existing cognitive impairment should be carefully assessed on an ongoing basis. Cognitive function should be assessed at least 24 hours following ECT, to avoid contamination by acute postictal effects. If confusion proves to be a problem, consideration should be given to switching from bilateral to unilateral ECT. None the less, Stoudemire *et al* (1991) found no significant difference in the cognitive outcome of elderly patients with depression treated with ECT or tricyclic antidepressant medication, and the detrimental effect of severe untreated depression on cognitive function far outweighs that of ECT (Wilkinson *et al*, 1993). ECT can be given to patients with dementia and depression without ill effect (Benbow, 1988; Liang *et al*, 1988) but they may be at increased risk of post-ECT delirium (Godber *et al*, 1987).

In conclusion:

- ECT is a safe and effective treatment for depression in elderly people.
- Special attention should be given to underlying physical illnesses because of the associated greater risks from anaesthesia.
- Regular assessment of cognitive function at least 24 hours after the administration of ECT is recommended.
- ECT technique may need to be modified, to minimise cognitive adverse effects (see Chapters 8 and 16).

The use of ECT as treatment for depression in pregnancy

It was thought that pregnancy protected women against depression. However, Watson *et al* (1984) found that 23% of all cases of postnatal depression started during pregnancy. In a cohort study involving 9028 women who completed four questionnaires, Evans *et al* (2001) showed that self-reported symptom scores for depression were higher in pregnancy than postnatally, and that the severity and nature of the depressed mood did not differ before and after childbirth.

A large number of reports show the efficacy of and very few complications from the use of ECT in all three trimesters of pregnancy (Oates, 1986; Wisner & Peril, 1988; Nurnberg, 1989; Ferrill *et al*, 1992; Miller, 1994; Walker & Swartz, 1994). This database does not exist for many of the newer antidepressants or atypical antipsychotics. There are also no studies on the potential for tetratogenicity of newer anti-depressants in combination with newer antipsychotics.

Miller (1994) reviewed 300 cases of ECT in pregnancy. Complications were noted in 9.3%. Many did not show any temporal relationship to the administration of ECT. The incidence of genetic malformations after ECT was also lower than seen in a historical control population (Nelson & Holmes, 1989).

Of the drugs used in anaesthesia for the administration of ECT, only anticholinergics are of concern. This is because they may increase the risk of regurgitation by lowering the oesophageal sphincter tone. The decision to use anticholinergics during anaesthesia should be made by the anaesthetist after weighing up the risks involved. If an anti-cholinergic is used, glycopyrrolate (marketed in UK as glycopyrronium bromide) is preferable because its placental transfer is more limited than that of atropine (Proakis & Harris, 1978; Abboud *et al*, 1983; Ferrill *et al*, 1992; Miller, 1994).

When administering ECT in pregnancy the following additions to current ECT practice are recommended (Heath & Yonkers, 2001):

- obstetric consultation before referral for ECT
- routine fetal heart monitoring before and after each individual treatment when gestational age is beyond the first trimester (obstetric consultation may suggest earlier monitoring in high-risk pregnancies)
- case-by-case consideration of intubation, because of the risk of regurgitation, particularly beyond the first trimester.

Obstetric consultation could confirm that the proposed ECT facility is appropriate in case an obstetric or neonatal complication arises (Ferrill *et al*, 1992; Miller, 1994) – facilities intending to use ECT in pregnant woman should have resources available to deal with obstetric and neonatal emergencies (Miller, 1994).

The place of ECT in the treatment of depressive illness during pregnancy will depend on the same kinds of balances described above for non-pregnant patients.

The use of ECT in children and adolescents for the treatment of depression

The first edition of *The ECT Handbook* included separate notes on the use of ECT for people under 18 years of age because of the considerable debate this topic aroused. It was noted that those aged 16–18 years were able to consent to and refuse treatment in just the same way as older people. For adolescents under 16, parental consent was required in England and Wales, but not in Scotland; even when consent was given by the patient and the parents, it was recommended that an independent second opinion be sought from a child and adolescent psychiatrist.

The use of ECT in children and adolescents remains controversial (Baker, 1995; Baldwin & Jones, 1998). There is very limited information about it and what there is is mostly in the form of single case reports or small collections of patients (Rey & Walter, 1997). There is a general consensus that ECT is an effective treatment for some mental disorders in adolescents and that the indications, response and unwanted side-effects are similar to those observed in adults (Rey & Walter, 1997; Walter & Rey, 1997). This conclusion has to be qualified because of lack of systemic evidence.

In a study involving child and adolescent psychiatrists in the USA, more than half the respondents said that they had minimal knowledge about the use of ECT in children and adolescents (Ghaziuddin *et al*, 2001). Of a sample of 125 child and adolescent psychiatrists identified in a mail survey in the UK, 79% had never used ECT (Parmar, 1993). A nationwide survey of all ECT clinics (National Health Service and private) in Scotland between 1997 and 1999 found no examples of ECT prescribed to people under 17 years old (Freeman *et al*, 2000). These findings confirm the rarity of the use of ECT with young people.

Short-term memory problems were reported in 22% of courses of ECT in a study by Walter & Rey (1997). A more recent study showed an absence of cognitive impairment on the long-term follow-up in adolescents treated with ECT (Cohen *et al*, 1997). That study, however, included only ten patients.

The following are recommended:

- ECT should be used with caution in young people because of the lack of evidence from RCTs.
- First-line use in young people should be very rare.
- For a person under 16, two independent opinions should be available from child and adolescent psychiatrists. One opinion from a child and adolescent psychiatrist is sufficient with 16- to 17- year olds, because there is more literature documenting the safety and efficacy of ECT for this age group.

- Because of reports of increased length of seizures and post-ECT convulsions, clinicians are advised to stop all non-essential medications used by the patient at the time of the course of ECT (Rey & Walter, 1997).
- Stimulus dosing should take into account the lower seizure threshold in young people (Cohen *et al*, 1997; Kellner *et al*, 1998). The previous edition of *The ECT Handbook* recommended initial treatment with a dose as low as 25 mC.
- Consent requires specific attention. Parents and the child should be involved whenever possible (Rey & Walter, 1997). Where it is not possible to obtain informed consent, ECT should be given only when the patient's life is at risk from suicide or physical debilitation because of depressive illness.

The need for continuation pharmacotherapy in the prevention of relapse following ECT

Given the current shift to using ECT for severe, recurrent and treatment-resistant depression, relapse after its use can be expected (Sackeim *et al*, 2001). The risk of relapse is high even when adequate extended pharma-cotherapy is provided (Grunhaus *et al*, 1990). SSRIs may play a role in relapse prevention (Lauritzen *et al*, 1996). There is no objective evidence for the clinical notion that continuation ECT is more effective than continuation medication (Wijkstra *et al*, 2000). Although no prospective trails are available, there are retrospective 'reviews' that support the use of continuation ECT and medication together and that suggest this is more effective in preventing relapse than antidepressants on their own (Gagne *et al*, 2000). There is an urgent need for research in this field.

For all patients, the first 4–6 months after successful ECT treatment is the time of highest risk of relapse. This should be clearly reflected in the arrangements for psychiatric supervision, as already recommended in the previous edition of *The ECT Handbook*.

The effect of ECT on cognitive function

Very few trials with comparative data about cognitive function could be found. The data that are available suggest the following:

- ECT can cause changes in both short-term anterograde and retrograde memory. It remains unclear how long this may persist.
- Variations in the method of ECT (e.g. bilateral versus unilateral, three times versus twice per week and high dose versus low dose) have an effect on cognitive function after ECT.
- There is little evidence from randomised studies that a sinusoidal waveform causes more memory impairment than brief-pulse ECT.

It has been shown that patients with a severe depressive illness have impaired cognitive function on recovery from an episode of illness even if not treated with ECT (Brodaty *et al*, 2001). There is evidence that ECT can cause persistent or permanent memory loss (Squire *et al*, 1981; Weiner *et al*, 1986; McElhiney *et al*, 1995; Sobin *et al*, 1995), which is difficult to distinguish from that caused by illness. Deficits are usually in recall of both autobiographical memory and 'public information' (knowledge of events in the world).

The more effective forms of ECT (i.e. higher-dose and bilateral ECT) cause more cognitive defects. Because each form of administering ECT has a risk–benefit ratio, it should be tailored to the specific clinical need of the patient.

We would therefore strongly recommend that the possibility of both short-term and long-term cognitive impairment is discussed with both the patient and the nearest relative, or an advocate if no relative is available. This should be clearly documented in the patient's notes.

Recommendations

Electroconvulsive therapy is a proven effective treatment for depression. It is a safe form of treatment even in the medically ill, the elderly and in pregnancy. There are benefits in using it in emergencies. It should not be relegated to a treatment of last resort. We would recommend that ECT be used in the treatment of depression using the following guidelines.

- As a first-line treatment for:
    - the emergency treatment of depression where a rapid definitive response is needed
    - patients with high suicidal risk
    - patients with severe psychomotor retardation and associated problems of eating and drinking or physical deterioration
    - a patient who suffers from treatment-resistant depression and who has responded to ECT in a previous episode of illness
    - patients who are pregnant, if there is concern about the teratogenic effects of antidepressants and antipsychotics
    - patients for whom it is the preferred choice of treatment and for whom there are strong clinical indications for its use.

- As a second-line treatment for:
    - patients with treatment-resistant depression
    - patients who experience severe side-effects from medication, limiting effective treatment
    - patients whose medical or psychiatric condition, in spite of adequate pharmacotherapy, has deteriorated to an extent that raises concern.

References

Abboud, I., Raya, J., Sadri, S., *et al* (1983) Fetal and maternal cardiovascular effects of atropine and glycopyrrolate. *Anesthesia and Analgesia*, **62**, 426–430.

Abrams, R. & Taylor, M. A. (1976) Catatonia: a prospective clinical study. *Archives of General Psychiatry*, **33**, 579–581.

Alexopoulos, G. S., Shamoian, C. J., Weiser, N., *et al* (1984) Medical problems of geriatric psychiatric patients and younger controls during electroconvulsive therapy. *Journal of the American Geriatrics Society*, **32**, 651–654.

American Psychiatric Association (1994) *Diagnostic and Statistical Manual of Mental Disorders* (4th edn) (DSM–IV). Washington, DC: APA.

Baker, T. (1995) ECT and young minds. *Lancet*, **345**, 65.

Baldwin, S. & Jones, Y. (1998) Is electroconvulsive therapy unsuitable for children and adolescents? *Adolescence*, **33**, 645–655.

Benbow, S. M. (1987) The use of electroconvulsive therapy in old age psychiatry. *International Journal of Geriatric Psychiatry*, **2**, 25–30.

Benbow, S. M. (1988) ECT for depression in dementia. *British Journal of Psychiatry*, **152**, 859.

Bidder, T. G., Strain, J. J. & Brundschwig, L. (1970) Bilateral and unilateral ECT: follow-up study and critique. *American Journal of Psychiatry*, **127**, 737–745.

Brodaty, H., Berle, D., Hicki, I., *et al* (2001) Side effects of ECT are mainly depressive phenomena and are independent of age. *Journal of Affective Disorders*, **66**, 327–345.

Buchan, H., Johnstone, E., McPherson, K., *et al* (1992) Who benefits from electroconvulsive therapy? Combined results of the Leicester and Northwick Park trials. *British Journal of Psychiatry*, **160**, 355–359.

Burke, W. J., Ruben, E. H., Zorumzki, C. F., *et al* (1987) Safety of ECT in geriatric psychiatry. *Journal of the American Geriatrics Society*, **35**, 516–521.

Burrows, G. D., Norman, T. R. & Judd, F. K. (1994) Definition and differential diagnosis of treatment resistant depression. *International Clinical Psychopharmacology*, **9** (suppl. 4), 5–10.

Bush, G., Fink, M., Petrides, G., *et al.* (1996*a*) Catatonia I. Rating scale and standardised examination. *Acta Psychiatrica Scandinavica*, **93**, 129–136.

Bush, G., Fink, M., Petrides, G., *et al.* (1996*b*) Catatonia II. Treatment with lorazepam and electroconvulsive therapy. *Acta Psychiatrica Scandinavica*, **93**, 137–143.

Cohen, D., Paillere-Marmot, M. & Basquin, M. (1997) Use of electroconvulsive therapy in adolescents. *Convulsive Therapy*, **13**, 25–31.

Devenand, D. P. & Kruger, R. B. (1994) Electroconvulsive therapy in the elderly. *Current Opinion in Psychiatry*, **7**, 359–364.

Eranti, S. V. & McLoughlin, D. M. (2003) Electroconvulsive therapy – state of the art. *British Journal of Psychiatry*, **182**, 8–9.

Evans, J., Heron, J., Francombe, H., *et al* (2001) Cohort study of depressed mood during pregnancy and after childbirth. *British Medical Journal*, **323**, 257–260.

Fava, M. & Davidson, K. G. (1996) Definition and epidemiology of treatment resistant depression. *Psychiatric Clinics of North America*, **19**, 179–200.

Ferrill, M. J., Kehoe, W. A. & Jacisin, J. J. (1992) ECT during pregnancy: physiologic and pharmacologic considerations. *Convulsive Therapy*, **8**, 186–200.

Folkerts, H. W., Micheal, N., Tolle, R., *et al* (1997) Electroconvulsive therapy vs. paroxetine in treatment resistant depression: a randomised study. *Acta Psychiatrica Scandinavica*, **96**, 334–342.

Freeman, C. P., Basson, J. V. & Crighton, A. (1978) Double-blind controlled trial of electroconvulsive therapy (ECT) and simulated ECT in depressive illness. *Lancet*, *i*, 738–740.

Freeman, C. P. L., Hendry, J. & Fergusson, G. (2000) *National Audit of Electroconvulsive Therapy in Scotland. Final Report.* Available at www.sean.org.uk/report/report00.php.

Fricchione, G. L. (1989) Catatonia: a new indication for benzodiazepines? *Biological Psychiatry*, **26**, 761–765.

Fricchione, G. L., Cassem, N. H., Hooberman, D., *et al* (1983) Intravenous lorazepam in neuroleptic-induced catatonia. *Journal of Clinical Psychopharmacology*, **3**, 338–342.

Gagne, G., Furman, M. J., Carpenter, L. L., *et al* (2000) Efficacy of continuation ECT and antidepressant drugs compared to long-term antidepressants alone in depressed patients. *American Journal of Psychiatry*, **157**, 1960–1965.

Gangadhar, B. N., Janakiramaiah, N., Subbakrishna, D. K., *et al* (1993) Twice versus thrice weekly ECT in melancholia: a double-blind prospective comparison. *Journal of Affective Disorders*, **27**, 273–278.

Gellenberg, A. J. (1977) Catatonic reactions to high-potency neuroleptic drugs. *Archives of General Psychiatry*, **34**, 947–950.

Ghaziuddin, N., Kaza, M., Ghazi, N., *et al* (2001) Electroconvulsive therapy for minors: experiences and attitudes of child psychiatrists and psychologists. *Journal of ECT*, **17**, 109–117.

Godber, C., Rosenvinge, H., Wilkinson, D., *et al* (1987) Depression in old age: prognosis after ECT. *International Journal of Geriatric Psychiatry*, **2**, 19–24.

Gregory, S., Shawcross, C. R. & Gill, D. (1985) The Nottingham ECT Study. A double-blind comparison of bilateral, unilateral and simulated ECT in depressive illness. *British Journal of Psychiatry*, **146**, 520–524.

Grunhaus, L., Pande, A. C. & Haskett, R. F. (1990) Full and abbreviated courses of maintenance electroconvulsive therapy. *Convulsive Therapy*, **6**, 130–138.

Heath, C. & Yonkers, K. A. (2001) Somatic treatments in depression: concerns during pregnancy and breastfeeding. In *Management of Psychiatric Disorders in Pregnancy* (eds K. Yonkers & B. Little). London: Arnold.

Heshe, J., Roder, E. & Theilgard, A. (1978) Unilateral and bilateral ECT. A psychiatric and psychological study of therapeutic effect and side effects. *Acta Psychiatrica Scandinavica Supplementum* (275), 1–180.

Hussain, S. S. (2002) *Electroconvulsive Therapy in Depressive Illness that has not Responded to Drug Treatment.* MPhil thesis, University of Edinburgh.

Janakiramaiah, N., Motreja, S., Gangadhar, B. N., *et al* (1998a) Once vs. three times weekly ECT in melancholia: a randomised control trial. *Acta Psychiatrica Scandinavica*, **98**, 316–320.

Janakiramaiah, N., Motreja, S., Gangadhar, B. N., *et al* (1998b) EEG seizure in bilateral ECT is different between low and high stimulus doses. *Clinical Electroencephalography*, **29**, 197–199.

Johnstone, E. C., Deakin, J. F., Lawler, P., *et al* (1980) The Northwick Park electroconvulsive therapy trial. *Lancet*, **ii**, 1317–1320.

Kellner, C. H., Monroe, J., Prichett, J., *et al* (1992) Weekly ECT in geriatric depression. *Convulsive Therapy*, **8**, 245–252.

Kellner, C. H., Beale, M. D. & Bernstein, H. J. (1998) Electroconvulsive therapy. In *Handbook of Child and Adolescent Psychiatry*, Vol. 6 (ed. C. D. Noshpitz), pp. 269–272. New York: Wiley.

Kindler, M., Shapira, B., Hadjez, J., *et al* (1991) Factors influencing response to bilateral electroconvulsive therapy in major depression. *Convulsive Therapy*, **7**, 245–254.

Liang, R. A., Lam, R. W. & Ancill, R. J. (1988) ECT in the treatment of mixed depression and dementia. *British Journal of Psychiatry*, **152**, 281–284.

Lambourn, J. & Gill, D. (1978) A controlled comparison of simulated and real ECT. *British Journal of Psychiatry*, **133**, 514–519.

Lauritzen, L., Odgaard, K., Clemmesen, L., *et al.* (1996) Relapse prevention by means of paroxetine in ECT treated patients with major depression: a comparison with imipramine and placebo in medium-term continuation therapy. *Acta Psychiatrica Scandinavica*, **94**, 241–251.

Lerer, B., Shapira, B., Calev, A., *et al* (1995) Antidepressant and cognitive effects of twice- versus three-times weekly ECT. *American Journal of Psychiatry*, **152**, 564–570.

Lock, T. (1995) Stimulus dosing. In *The ECT Handbook. The Second Report of the Royal College of Psychiatrists' Special Committee on ECT* (Council Report CR39) (ed. C. P. Freeman), pp. 72–87. London: Royal College of Psychiatrists.

Lock, T. & McCulloch, J. (1991) Local glucose utilization after chronic electroconvulsive shock: implications for mode of action of electroconvulsive therapy. *Journal of Psychopharmacology*, **5**, 111–119.

Mann, S. C., Caroff, S. N., Bleier, H. R., *et al* (1986) Lethal catatonia. *American Journal of Psychiatry*, **143**, 1374–1381.

McCall, W. V., Farah, B. A., Reboussin, D., *et al* (1995) Comparison of the efficacy of titrated, moderate-dose and fixed, high-dose right unilateral ECT in elderly patients. *American Journal of Geriatric Psychiatry*, **3**, 317–324.

McCall, W. V., Reboussin, D. M., Weiner, R. D., *et al* (2000) Titrated moderately suprathreshold vs. fixed high-dose unilateral electroconvulsive therapy: acute antidepressant and cognitive effects. *Archives of General Psychiatry*, **57**, 438–444.

McElhiney, M. C., Moody, B. J., Steif, B. L., *et al* (1995) Autobiographical memory and mood: effects of electroconvulsive therapy. *Neuropsychology*, **9**, 501–517.

Miller, L. J. (1994) Use of electroconvulsive therapy during pregnancy. *Hospital and Community Psychiatry*, **45**, 444–450.

Mulsant, B. H., Rosen, J., Thornton, J., *et al* (1991) A prospective naturalistic study of electroconvulsive therapy in late life depression. *Journal of Geriatric Psychiatry and Neurology*, **4**, 3–13.

Nelson, K. & Holmes, L. B. (1989) Malformations due to presumed spontaneous mutations in newborn infants. *New England Journal of Medicine*, **320**, 19–23.

Nierenberg, A. A. & Amsterdam, J. D. (1990) Treatment-resistant depression: definition and treatment approaches. *Journal of Clinical Psychiatry*, **51** (suppl.), 39–47 (discussion 48–50).

Nurnberg, H. G. (1989) An overview of somatic treatment of psychoses during pregnancy and postpartum. *General Hospital Psychiatry*, **11**, 328–338.

Oates, M. R. (1986) The treatment of psychiatric disorders in pregnancy and the puerperium. *Clinics in Obstetrics and Gynaecology*, **13**, 385–395.

O'Leary, D., Gill, D., Gregory, S., *et al* (1995) Which depressed patients respond to ECT? The Nottingham results. *Journal of Affective Disorders*, **33**, 245–250.

Parmar, R. (1993) Attitudes of child psychiatrists to electroconvulsive therapy. *Psychiatric Bulletin*, **17**, 12–13.

Pataki, J., Zervas, I. M. & Jandorf, L. (1992) Catatonia in a university inpatient service (1985–1990). *Convulsive Therapy*, **8**, 162–173.

Pearlman, C. (1991) Electroconvulsive therapy: current concepts. *General Hospital Psychiatry*, **13**, 128–137.

Porter, R. & Ferrier, N. (1999) Emergency treatment of depression. *Advances in Psychiatric Treatment*, **5**, 3–10.

Post, R. M., Uhde, T. W., Rubinow, D. R., *et al* (1987) Differential time course of antidepressant effects after sleep deprivation, ECT, and carbamazepine: clinical and theoretical implications. *Psychiatry Research*, **22**, 11–19.

Proakis, A. G. & Harris, G. B. (1978) Comparative penetration of glycopyrrolate and atropine across the blood–brain and placental barriers in anaesthetized dogs. *Anaesthesiology*, **48**, 339–344.

Prudic, J., Sackeim, H. A. & Devanand, D. P. (1990) Medication resistance and clinical response to ECT. *Psychiatry Research*, **31**, 287–296.

Prudic, J., Haskett, R. F., Mulsant, B., *et al* (1996) Resistance to antidepressant medications and short-term clinical response to ECT. *American Journal of Psychiatry*, **153**, 985–992.

Rey, J. M. & Walter, G. (1997) Half a century of ECT use in young people. *American Journal of Psychiatry*, **154**, 595–602.

Rice, E. H., Sombrotto, L. B., Markowitz, J. C., *et al* (1994) Cardiovascular morbidity in high-risk patients during ECT. *American Journal of Psychiatry*, **151**, 1637–1641.

Robin, A. & de Tissera, S. (1982) A double blind controlled comparison of the therapeutic effects of low and high energy electroconvulsive therapies. *British Journal of Psychiatry*, **141**, 357–366.

Rodger, C. R., Scott, A. I. & Whalley, L. J. (1994) Is there a delay in the onset of the antidepressant effect of electroconvulsive therapy? *British Journal of Psychiatry*, **164**, 106–109.

Rosebush, P. I., Hildebrand, A. M., Furlong, B. G., *et al* (1990) Catatonic syndrome in a general psychiatric population: frequency, clinical presentation, and response to lorazepam. *Journal of Clinical Psychiatry*, **51**, 357–362.

Sackeim, H. A. (1992) The cognitive effects of electroconvulsive therapy. In *Cognitive Disorders: Pathophysiology and Treatment* (eds L. J. Thal *et al*), pp. 183–228. New York: Marcel Dekker.

Sackeim, H. A. (2001) The definition and meaning of treatment-resistant depression. *Journal of Clinical Psychiatry*, **62** (suppl. 16), 10–17.

Sackeim, H. A., Prudic, J., Devanand, D. P., *et al* (1993) Effects of stimulus intensity and electrode placement on the efficacy and cognitive effects of electroconvulsive therapy. *New England Journal of Medicine*, **328**, 839–846.

Sackeim, H. A., Luber, B., Moeller, J. R., *et al* (2000*a*) Electrophysiological correlates of the adverse cognitive effects of electroconvulsive therapy. *Journal of ECT*, **16**, 110–120.

Sackeim, H. A., Prudic, J., Devanand, D. P., *et al* (2000*b*) A prospective, randomised, double-blind comparison of bilateral and right unilateral electroconvulsive therapy at different stimulus intensities. *Archives of General Psychiatry*, **57**, 425–434.

Sackeim, H. A., Haskett, R. F., Mulsant, B. H., *et al* (2001) Continuation pharmaco-therapy in the prevention of relapse following electroconvulsive therapy: a randomized controlled trial. *Journal of the American Medical Association*, **285**, 1299–1307.

Shapira, B., Tubi, N., Drexler, H., *et al* (1998) Cost and benefit in the choice of ECT schedule. Twice versus three times weekly ECT. *British Journal of Psychiatry*, **172**, 44–48.

Sobin, C., Sackeim, H. A., Prudic, J., *et al* (1995) Predictors of retrograde amnesia following ECT. *American Journal of Psychiatry*, **152**, 995–1001.

Sobin, C., Prudic, J., Devanand, D. P., *et al* (1996) Who responds to electroconvulsive therapy? A comparison of effective and ineffective forms of treatment. *British Journal of Psychiatry*, **169**, 322–328.

Souery, D., Amsterdam, J., de Montigny, C., *et al* (1999) Treatment resistant depression: methodological overview and operational criteria. *European Psychopharmacology*, **9**, 83–91.

Squire, L. R., Slater, P. C. & Miller, P. L. (1981) Retrograde amnesia and bilateral electroconvulsive therapy. Long-term follow-up. *Archives of General Psychiatry*, **38**, 89–95.

Stoudemire, A., Hill, C. D., Morris, R., *et al* (1991) Cognitive outcome following tricyclic and electroconvulsive treatment of depression in the elderly. *American Journal of Psychiatry*, **148**, 1336–1349.

Swartz, C., Morrow, V., Surles, L., *et al* (2001) Long-term outcome after ECT for catatonia depression. *Journal of ECT*, **17**, 180–183.

Taylor, M. A. (1990) Catatonia: a review of a behavioural neurologic syndrome. *Neuropsychiatry, Neuropsychology and Behavioral Neurology*, **3**, 48–72.

Tew, J. D., Mulsant, B. H., Haskett, R. F., *et al* (1999) Acute efficacy of ECT in the treatment of major depression in the old-old. *American Journal of Psychiatry*, **156**, 1865–1870.

UK ECT Review Group (2003) Efficacy and safety of electro-convulsive therapy in depressive disorders: a systematic review and meta-analysis. *Lancet*, **361**, 799–808.

Ungvari, G. A., Leung, C. M., Wong, M. K., *et al* (1994) Benzodiazepines in the treatment of catatonic syndrome. *Acta Psychiatrica Scandinavica*, **89**, 285–288.

Vieweg, R. & Shawcross, C. R. (1998) Trial to determine any difference between two and three times a week ECT in the rate of recovery from depression. *Journal of Mental Health*, **7**, 403–409.

Walker, R. & Swartz, C. M. (1994) Electroconvulsive therapy during high-risk pregnancy. *General Hospital Psychiatry*, **16**, 348–353.

Walter, G. & Rey, M. (1997) An epidemiological study of the use of ECT in adolescents. *Journal of the American Academy of Child and Adolescent Psychiatry*, **36**, 809–815.

Watson, J. P., Elliot, S. A., Rugg, A. J., *et al* (1984) Psychiatric disorder in pregnancy and the first postnatal year. *British Journal of Psychiatry*, **144**, 453–462.

Weiner, R. D., Rogers, H. J., Davidson, J. R., *et al* (1986) Effects of stimulus parameters on cognitive side effects. *Annals of the New York Academy of Sciences*, **462**, 315–325.

West, E. D. (1981) Electric convulsion therapy in depression: a double blind controlled trial. *British Medical Journal*, **282**, 355–357.

Wijkstra, J., Nolen, W., Algra, A., *et al* (2000) Relapse prevention in major depressive disorder after successful ECT: a literature review and a naturalistic case series. *Acta Psychiatrica Scandinavica*, **102**, 454–460.

Wilkinson, A. M., Anderson, D. N. & Peters, S. (1993) Age and the effects of ECT. *International Journal of Geriatric Psychiatry*, **8**, 401–406.

Wilson, I. C., Vernon, J. T., Guin, T., *et al* (1963) A controlled study of treatments of depression. *Journal of Neuropsychiatry*, **4**, 331–337.

Wisner, K. L. & Peril, J. M. (1988) Psychopharmacologic agents and electroconvulsive therapy. In *Psychiatric Consultation in Childbirth Settings: Parent and Child-Orientated Approaches* (ed. R. E. L. Cohn), pp. 165–206. New York: Plenum.

Zielinski, R. J., Roose, S. P., Devanand, D. P., *et al* (1993) Cardiovascular complications of ECT in depressed patients with cardiac disease. *American Journal of Psychiatry*, **150**, 904–909.

CHAPTER 3

The use of ECT in the treatment of mania

Andrew M. Whitehouse

Some of the earliest case reports of the efficacy of convulsive therapy concerned patients who were manic. Similar reports were made soon after the introduction of electrical induction in the 1940s. In reviewing these papers Mukherjee *et al* (1994) noted that the proportion of patients showing remission or marked clinical improvement varied between 63% and 84%.

Empirical results

In 1977 the Royal College of Psychiatrists commented that 'there are no satisfactory controlled studies of the use of ECT in mania'. At that time there was one recently conducted study (McCabe, 1976) comparing patients with mania treated with ECT with an untreated matched control group from a period when ECT was unavailable. The ECT-treated group had a better outcome and shorter hospital stay. These two groups were then compared with a matched group treated with chlorpromazine (McCabe & Norris, 1977). Of the 28 patients treated with chlorpromazine 18 were responders, compared with all 28 patients treated with ECT. All 10 chlorpromazine non-responders went on to receive ECT and responded. This study therefore suggests ECT to be a superior treatment to chlorpromazine.

Retrospective studies

There have been five further retrospective studies. Thomas & Reddy (1982) found ECT, chlorpromazine and lithium to be equally effective. Black *et al* (1987) found a significantly greater proportion of ECT-treated patients improved markedly than lithium-treated patients. The other three studies, with no comparison groups, found marked clinical improvement or remission in 56–78% of patients (Alexander *et al*, 1988; Stromgren, 1988; Mukherjee & Debsikdar, 1992).

Prospective studies

There have been three prospective studies of the efficacy of ECT in mania. Small et al (1988) randomised 34 patients hospitalised with mania to ECT or lithium carbonate. Unilateral ECT was initially prescribed but with the option of switching to bilateral ECT. The details of stimulus dosing were not provided. After the first six patients received unilateral ECT with little or no benefit, or even a worsening of their condition, the study design was changed so that bilateral ECT was administered from the beginning. ECT was given three times weekly. Both the ECT and lithium groups received concomitant antipsychotic medication. When the ECT treatment was completed, patients were prescribed prophylactic lithium carbonate. Over an 8-week period, ratings of observers indicated that the ECT-treated patients improved more than those treated with lithium carbonate.

Mukherjee et al (1988) examined the effectiveness of ECT in 20 patients with mania who had proved treatment resistant to pharmaco-therapy of at least 3 weeks' duration. The patients were randomised to receive left unilateral ECT, right unilateral ECT, bilateral ECT or a lithium and haloperidol combination (five patients in each group). Empirical measurement of the seizure threshold was conducted at the start of ECT, and thereafter the stimulus exceeded the seizure threshold by 150%. Fifty-nine per cent of the ECT-treated patients were responders, compared with none of the small group of patients receiving pharmaco-therapy. No difference in outcome was found between unilateral and bilateral ECT.

Sikdar et al (1994) were the only group to compare actual ECT with simulated or 'sham' ECT. In this double-blind controlled study, 30 patients who fulfilled the DSM–III–R criteria for a manic episode (American Psychiatric Association, 1987) were randomised to an experimental group or a control group. The experimental group received eight bilateral ECT treatments in addition to 600 mg chlorpromazine. After a patient had received six ECT treatments, the dose of chlor-promazine could be changed, or another antipsychotic could be prescribed in its place. The control group received eight simulated ECT treatments and their medication was managed in an identical way to that of the experimental group. At the end of the study 12 patients in the ECT group were completely recovered, compared with only one patient in the simulated ECT group. There was a significantly greater decrease on the Mania Rating Scale (Bech et al, 1979) in the ECT group compared with the simulated group after the second, fourth, sixth and eighth ECT treatments ($P<0.001$). Eleven patients in the simulated ECT group required an increase in antipsychotic medication compared with two patients in the ECT group, which is a significant difference ($P <0.05$). The patients receiving real ECT also had a significantly shorter duration of illness than the simulated ECT group. Sikdar *et al* (1994) commented that their findings 'demonstrate that a combination of ECT and a moderate dose of a neuroleptic is extremely effective in rapidly aborting an acute episode of mania'. They concluded that their results 'highlight the fact that ECT can be recommended for any manic patient, irrespective of the severity or the duration of the illness'.

Electrode placement

Controversy exists about the relative efficacy of unilateral and bilateral ECT. As indicated above, Small *et al* (1988) found that the first six patients with mania receiving unilateral ECT failed to respond in their comparison of ECT and lithium carbonate. In a retrospective study Small *et al* (1985) had earlier identified the characteristics of patients who failed to respond to unilateral ECT but subsequently responded to bilateral ECT. This group of 25 patients was compared with a similar number of patients who responded to unilateral ECT. Both groups comprised patients with manic symptoms, but a variety of diagnoses. Although there was no excess of patients diagnosed as suffering from mania in the group that switched, there was a significant excess of manic symptoms in this group ($P<0.005$). Small *et al* (1985) concluded that 'patients who exhibit significant symptoms of mania and who do not respond to right unilateral ECT, can benefit from bilateral treatment'. They went on to say that 'in all probability such patients should receive bilateral treatment from the beginning'.

Mukherjee *et al* (1988) found no difference between unilateral and bilateral ECT in patients with mania, but the study lacked the statistical power to compare the treatments because of the small sample size.

These studies of the efficacy of unilateral ECT were conducted before it was clearly established that electrical dose was an important determinant of the efficacy of unilateral ECT in depressive illness. There has never been a controlled comparison of, say, moderate- or high-dose unilateral ECT with moderate-dose bilateral ECT. It is not known therefore whether unilateral ECT is for some unknown fundamental reason less efficacious than bilateral ECT, or whether it can approximate the efficacy of bilateral ECT if it is given at an optimal dose. Where the speed of response is critical, for example in life-threatening illness, it may therefore be wise to prescribe bilateral ECT from the outset.

Mode of action

A number of theories regarding the mechanism of action of the antimanic effect of ECT have been proposed. Mukherjee (1989) stated that 'the standard view has been that the elicitation of a generalised tonic–clonic seizure of sufficient duration is critical to the therapeutic effects of ECT', and went on to discuss two alternative hypotheses. The first relates to the fact that seizure threshold rises during a course of ECT, and it is this activation of brain inhibitory processes that Mukherjee proposed could be responsible for the antimanic effect. In support of this hypothesis Mukherjee (1989) demonstrated that the proportional increase in seizure threshold was significantly greater in patients with mania who responded to ECT than in non-responders (P <0.05). He discussed the possibility of increased transmission of gamma-aminobutyric acid (GABA) and endogenous opioid peptides being involved in the inhibitory process. Mukherjee's (1989) second hypothesis was that the antimanic effect of ECT is related to the reduction of cortical perfusion that occurs during a course of ECT, and he demonstrated a strong association between an antimanic response and this decrease in cortical perfusion. Sikdar *et al* (1994) have suggested the possibility that ECT causes changes in the blood–brain barrier that increase the transport of antipsychotic medication into the central nervous system.

Recommendations

Electroconvulsive therapy has been shown to be an efficacious treatment in mania. The Consensus Group (see Chapter 1) concluded that the treatment of choice for the general case of mania was a mood-stabilising drug plus an antipsychotic drug. ECT may be considered for severe mania associated with life-threatening physical exhaustion or treatment resistance, that is, mania that has not responded to the treatment of choice.

The optimal technique for the administration of unilateral ECT has not been established in mania, but the bilateral placement may be preferred, particularly in life-threatening illness.

References

Alexander, R. C., Salmon, M., Ionescu-Pioggia, M., *et al* (1988) Convulsive therapy in the treatment of mania: McLean Hospital 1973–1986. *Convulsive Therapy*, **4**, 115–125.

American Psychiatric Association (1987) *Diagnostic and Statistical Manual of Mental Disorders* (3rd edn, revised) (DSM–III–R). Washington, DC: APA.

Bech, P., Bolwig, T. G., Kramp, P., *et al* (1979) The Bech–Rafaelsen Mania Scale and Hamilton Depression Scale. *Acta Psychiatrica Scandinavica*, **59**, 420–430.

Black, D. W., Winokur, G. & Nasrallah, A. (1987) A naturalistic study of electro-convulsive therapy versus lithium in 460 patients. *Journal of Clinical Psychiatry*, **48**, 132–139.

McCabe, M. S. (1976) ECT in the treatment of mania: a controlled study. *American Journal of Psychiatry*, **133**, 688–691.

McCabe, M. S. & Norris, B. (1977) ECT versus chlorpromazine in mania. *Biological Psychiatry*, **12**, 245–254.

Mukherjee, S. (1989) Mechanisms of the anti-manic effect of electroconvulsive therapy. *Convulsive Therapy*, **5**, 227–243.

Mukherjee, S. & Debsikdar, V. (1992) Unmodified electroconvulsive therapy of acute mania: a retrospective naturalistic study. *Convulsive Therapy*, **8**, 5–11.

Mukherjee, S., Sackheim, H. A. & Lee, C. (1988) Unilateral ECT in the treatment of manic episodes. *Convulsive Therapy*, **4**, 74–80.

Mukherjee, S., Sackheim, H. A. & Schnur, D. B. (1994) Electroconvulsive therapy of acute manic episodes: a review of 50 years' experience. *American Journal of Psychiatry*, **151**, 169–176.

Royal College of Psychiatrists (1977) Memorandum on the use of electroconvulsive therapy. *British Journal of Psychiatry*, **131**, 261–272.

Sikdar, S., Kulhara, P., Avasthi, A., *et al* (1994) Combined chlorpromazine and electroconvulsive therapy in mania. *British Journal of Psychiatry*, **164**, 806–810.

Small, J. G., Small, I. F., Milstein, V., *et al* (1985) Manic symptoms: an indication for bilateral ECT. *Biological Psychiatry*, **20**, 125–134.

Small, J. G., Klapper, M. H., Kellams, J. J., *et al* (1988) Electroconvulsive treatment compared with lithium in the management of manic states. *Archives of General Psychiatry*, **45**, 727–732.

Stromgren, L. S. (1988) Electroconvulsive therapy in Aarhus, Denmark, in 1984: its application in non-depressive disorders. *Convulsive Therapy*, **4**, 306–313.

Thomas, J. & Reddy, B. (1982) The treatment of mania: a retrospective evaluation of the effects of ECT, chlorpromazine, and lithium. *Journal of Affective Disorders*, **4**, 85–92.

CHAPTER 4

The use of ECT in the treatment of schizophrenia and catatonia

Christopher F. Fear

From its beginning in 1938 through the 1950s, ECT enjoyed considerable popularity for the treatment of schizophrenia. As one of very few available treatments, it appeared to offer rapid alleviation of psychotic symptoms, particularly in the acutely ill, and was said to be without significant risks. Nevertheless, the availability of antipsychotic drugs from 1953, together with increasing opposition to the use of ECT, led to its gradual decline through the 1960s and 1970s (Fink, 2001). A resurgence of interest in the 1980s concerning its use to augment the action of drugs in those resistant to neuroleptics was eclipsed with the arrival of atypical neuroleptics, particularly clozapine, for the pharmacotherapy of treatment-resistant schizophrenia. The finding that a proportion of patients have symptoms that fail to respond to clozapine has prompted investigation of combining this drug with ECT. In addition, many psychiatrists see ECT as the treatment of choice for catatonic schizophrenia.

It is remarkable that, despite being available for more than 60 years, there are few good-quality controlled trials of ECT for schizophrenia. This has not been rectified since the publication of the previous edition of *The ECT Handbook* (1995), but a number of excellent reviews of the available evidence have become available (Johns & Thompson, 1995; Krueger & Sackeim, 1995; Fink & Sackeim, 1996; Lehman *et al*, 1998). These were supplemented by a systematic review as part of the Cochrane Collaboration (Tharyan, 1996/2001). The present chapter constitutes a substantial revision of the earlier guidance to take account of these appraisals of the use of ECT in schizophrenia.

Efficacy

A comparison of real ECT against 'sham' ECT is the most rigorous method of establishing efficacy, comparable to a pharmaceutical placebo-controlled trial. In sham ECT the control group undergoes the full ECT procedure with the exception of the stimulus, controlling for all extraneous influences on outcome. The design was developed in the 1950s, and it often included a group who received a subconvulsive stimulus. These studies are fraught with ethical and methodological difficulties and few have been published since 1965. Moreover, a lack of operationalised diagnostic criteria, compounded by an overinclusive approach to schizophrenia in the USA, often resulting in the mis-diagnosis of affective psychoses, makes many of these early studies difficult to interpret. It is perhaps surprising, therefore, that it is primarily upon the results of these early studies that the American Psychiatric Association's Work Group on Schizophrenia based its assertion that ECT treatment gives a 50–70% improvement in psychosis and return to work in patients who have been ill for less than one year (American Psychiatric Association, 1997).

Krueger & Sackeim (1995) reviewed all four studies of ECT versus sham or subconvulsive ECT published between 1953 and 1964, one of which demonstrated the benefit of ECT over subconvulsive therapy. None found a therapeutic advantage for ECT over general anaesthesia alone. These studies can reasonably be criticised for their lack of diagnostic criteria and use of mixed samples of both chronic and acute psychotic presentations. It was not until the 1980s that this area was re-examined using a more rigorous approach, perhaps because of the ethical issues involved, together with the complexity of the study design, reflected in smaller sample sizes. The later studies used the Present State Examination or Research Diagnostic Criteria to classify their patients, and all three found ECT to be superior to sham ECT. It seems likely that the exclusion of chronic schizophrenia explains the different findings from earlier studies. Further, concurrent neuroleptic medication may have improved outcomes by enhancing the efficacy of ECT (see below). Sadly, none of the studies included medium- or long-term follow-up, so that the duration of improvement is not clear. Similar conclusions have been drawn by other authors (see Johns & Thompson, 1995; Fink & Sackeim, 1996; Lehman *et al*, 1998).

Under the auspices of the Cochrane Schizophrenia Group, Tharyan (1996/2001) reviewed all trials of ECT to determine whether treatment 'results in meaningful benefit with regard to global improvement, hospitalisation, changes in mental state, behaviour and functioning in those with schizophrenia'. Studies were identified using electronic searches and principal authors were contacted to obtain source data and details of other studies, published or unpublished. The review included only randomised controlled trials in which ECT was compared with placebo, sham ECT, antipsychotics and non-pharmacological inter-ventions (psychotherapy, social case-work, milieu therapy, etc.). The studies were examined by two reviewers, who assigned them to categories according to the Cochrane Collaboration Handbook, and only those that satisfied A or B quality standards were included. Of 36 studies considered, 12 were included, only one of which was assigned A quality. Exclusions were the result of inappropriate control groups (10), lack of or improper randomisation (12), both (1) or mixed diagnostic groups (1). All studies considered related either to schizophrenic or schizophreniform disorders. Data were extracted from the papers and subjected to statistical analyses, including odds ratios and confidence intervals for binary data, and numbers needed to treat. Nonparametric data were excluded. An advantage was found for ECT over placebo and sham ECT on the basis of ratings on the Clinical Global Improvement (CGI) scale and Brief Psychiatric Rating Scale (BPRS). ECT resulted in earlier improvement in BPRS scores which was maintained at 6 weeks after treatment. Limited data suggested that there were fewer relapses in the short term with ECT and that discharge from hospital was more likely, but 'sparse' data showed no evidence that the early improvement was maintained over 6–24 months.

In conclusion, there is evidence to support the efficacy of ECT in the short-term treatment of schizophrenic symptoms but no evidence to show that the effects are maintained in the medium to long term. The Cochrane review concluded that 'the lack of well randomised prospective trials and fundamental limitations in research design, methodology and reporting of trials, suggest that the widespread use of ECT as a treatment for those with schizophrenia in some parts of the world ... lacks a firm research base' (Tharyan, 1996/2001, p. 10).

ECT versus neuroleptics

There is a signal lack of trial data comparing ECT with neuroleptics. Three studies included in the Cochrane review compared ECT directly with neuroleptics. The review reports conflicting results, noting initially that 'when ECT is directly compared with antipsychotic drug treatment, the result is equivocal, but the trend favours the latter' (Tharyan, 1996/2000, p. 8); but later, 'ECT given alone is significantly less effective than antipsychotic medication over several outcomes, even in the short term' (p. 9). Patients on antipsychotic medication were more likely than those receiving ECT to be discharged from hospital. One study that compared ECT with psychoanalytical psychotherapy gave equivocal results, with a trend favouring ECT in both the short and medium term. The addition of neuroleptics to the psychotherapy group resulted in a significant advantage over ECT in the short term with a continued trend at 2-year follow-up.

Other authors have been less confused in their appraisal. The consensus view is that studies favour antipsychotic drug treatment over ECT in both the short and medium term (Johns & Thompson, 1995; Krueger & Sackeim, 1995; Fink & Sackeim, 1996; Lehman *et al*,

1998), although Krueger & Sackeim (1995, p. 514) assess these results as being limited 'in fundamental aspects of clinical trial methodology, particularly the reliability and validity of diagnosis, the nature of assignment to treatment groups, and the blindness and reliability of clinical evaluations'.

ECT combined with neuroleptics

Studies examining whether additional benefit is obtained from ECT plus neuroleptics as compared with neuroleptics or ECT alone have again run into considerable methodological problems, including questionable adequacy of pharmacotherapy, blindness and randomisation. Nine studies have been published to date, eight involving typical neuroleptics and considered in published reviews. The results suggest that the addition of ECT to neuroleptic treatment improves outcome in the short term in terms of number improved but without any evidence for an increased speed of response (Klapheke, 1993; Krueger & Sackeim, 1995). Four of these studies satisfied Cochrane inclusion criteria, and these showed a non-significant trend in favour of ECT plus antipsychotics with no data comparing discharge or relapse rates. Tharyan (1996/2001, p. 10) concluded that the 'results of trials most strongly favouring ECT in the short term ... suggest a role for the addition of ECT in those who show a limited response to antipsychotic medication'.

Using a more rigorous design, a recent study randomised 36 patients with operationally defined schizophrenia into three equal groups to receive thrice-weekly bilateral, unilateral non-dominant or sham ECT with concurrent haloperidol (Sarita *et al*, 1998). Subjects were rated by an independent psychiatrist, blind to treatment group, using the BPRS, CGI and a rating scale for extrapyramidal side-effects (EPSE). No therapeutic advantage was found for combined ECT and neuroleptics, whereas the ECT groups performed worse than the sham ECT group on memory tests 4 weeks after treatment. This study, despite its small sample size, is sounder in its design than many of those demonstrating a benefit for combined treatment and merits replication.

There is a single report of a case series in which the atypical neuroleptic risperidone was combined with ECT for the treatment of aggression in schizophrenia (Hirose *et al*, 2001). Ten male patients were given risperidone 5–9 mg daily together with 1 or 2 weeks of ECT five times per week. The authors claimed efficacy based on BPRS ratings but their data must be treated with circumspection because there were no controls or blinding of the raters and the small sample size. Finally, a novel use for ECT in combination with clozapine for acute schizophrenia has been reported by James & Gray (1999), who gave a course of 12 ECT sessions to six patients with treatment-resistant schizophrenia at the start of a course of concomitant clozapine. A 32% improvement on the BPRS at week 6 was seen as a rapid treatment response in patients who by then had sufficient insight to comply with blood testing and tablet taking. The mechanism and implication of this research bear further consideration.

Treatment resistance

Claims for the efficacy of ECT in treatment-resistant schizophrenia would perhaps best be described as a triumph of anecdote over empiricism. None of the studies considered by the Cochrane review met criteria for inclusion because, as asserted by Krueger & Sackeim (1995, p. 523), 'we have yet to have a double-blind, random assignment study contrasting the efficacy of ECT and neuroleptic treatment with continued neuroleptic treatment alone in medication-resistant schizophrenic patients'. The eight papers reviewed by them (which reported 'largely impressionistic observations', p. 523) suggested that, in a small minority of patients with chronic treatment-resistant schizophrenia, there may be a dramatic improvement, probably in patients with an affective component to their illness. Whether these are simply patients whose concurrent acute depression has been lost within their negative symptoms or whether there is a benefit to the schizophrenia per se is impossible to untangle, but there is little evidence for ECT alone improving chronic schizophrenia (Christison *et al*, 1991). There may be a benefit for patients with relatively short-term resistant illness but the data do not bear close scrutiny.

With the advent of atypical neuroleptic treatments, there has been less interest in the possible benefits of adding ECT to conventional neuroleptic treatment. Most pharmacotherapeutic algorithms indicate clozapine treatment for patients who are deemed 'treatment resistant' to adequate trials of two different classes of antipsychotic drugs (Lehman *et al*, 1998). Over the past decade there has been a growth of interest in ECT given in addition to atypical neuroleptics for patients with schizophrenia that has proved resistant to treatment with both conventional neuroleptics and clozapine. There has been some recent work from a group of researchers at the Srinakharinwirot University, Thailand, who have undertaken comparatively large open (Chanpattana *et al*, 1999*a*), randomised (Chanpattana, 2000) and randomised, blind (Chanpattana *et al*, 1999*b*) studies of ECT in combination with typical neuroleptics for medication-resistant schizophrenia. The studies suggest a benefit for combination therapy in the short term as well as for continuation and maintenance.

Electroconvulsive therapy was first recognised as a possible adjunct to clozapine treatment in 1991, with a case report of the administration of one treatment to a man with schizophrenia who was unresponsive to an 800 mg daily dose of clozapine (Masiar & Johns, 1991). Although the effects were not good, with two delayed seizures occurring 4 and 6 days after treatment, and no clinical improvement, other case reports followed. Reviewers have interpreted the results in remarkably different ways. Considering the same studies, two reviews have found no evidence that ECT enhances or hastens the response to clozapine (Krueger & Sackeim, 1995; Barnes *et al*, 1996), while one has suggested beneficial outcomes (Fink, 1998). Case reports continue to appear, most of which are positive (Benatov *et al*, 1996; Bhatia *et al*, 1998; Kales *et al*, 1999). A recent review of the literature (Kupchik *et al*, 2000) found reports of a total of 36 patients treated with combined ECT and clozapine for neuroleptic-resistant schizophrenia. Of these, 24 (67%) were reported to have responded, with a 16.6% incidence of adverse effects, including seizure prolongation, transient hypertension, sinus tachycardia, and supraventricular tachycardia in one patient whose seizure induction had been augmented with caffeine. Sadly, the authors' conclusions that this combination is effective and safe cannot be supported by any form of clinical trial.

In summary, while there are a tantalising number of case reports, most of which suggest a benefit from combining ECT with neuroleptics for treatment-resistant schizophrenic symptoms, the evidence base is too small and unreliable to allow conclusions to be drawn regarding its benefit, or otherwise. Resorting to this approach with patients for whom all other therapeutic opportunities have been exhausted is understandable and current evidence suggests that it is without major complications.

Maintenance ECT

The best time at which to end a course of ECT is uncertain and relapse is an ever-present concern. In a study of major depression, 50% of patients who responded to a course of ECT relapsed within a year, 79% of them within the first 4 months (Sackeim *et al*, 1990); no comparable data exist for schizophrenia. Early studies supported the use of maintenance ECT (mECT) for patients with schizophrenia who had responded to acute treatment. In one study, 12% of 57 patients who agreed to have maintenance ECT relapsed over a 5-year period, compared with 79% of the 153 patients who declined (Karliner & Wehrheim, 1965). These studies are unreliable as there are problems of design and diagnostic validity, as discussed previously. In considering recent studies, the distinction between continuation ECT (cECT), occurring within 6 months of acute treatment, and mECT, given beyond the 6-month point, as defined by the American Psychiatric Association Task

Force on ECT(1990), has been disregarded. In practice most studies blur this definition so that it seems of little value.

Stiebel (1995) retrospectively examined the notes of nine patients with schizophrenia ($n = 3$), schizoaffective disorder ($n = 2$) or affective disorder ($n = 4$) who received mECT from the University of Minnesota Hospital. Patients in the schizophrenia/schizoaffective group received up to four mECT treatments per month for 9–17 months after acute treatment and were reported to have made substantial recoveries which were sustained during the maintenance period, but relapsed after cessation of mECT. No significant adverse events were reported. A similar retrospective case review, this time at the University of Southern California, reported on 57 patients, three of whom had schizophrenia, who received mECT for 6–8 months (Kramer, 1999). The clinical characteristics of the patients are poorly reported but two were assessed to have been 'much improved', while one was 'partially improved'. The limitations of both studies are obvious and concurrent pharmaco-therapies were not recorded.

The only prospective series have been reported by Chanpattana and colleagues. In a pilot study of cECT 12 patients with schizophrenia who had responded to ECT were treated, neuroleptic free, with bilateral ECT for 6 months. The treatment regimen was weekly for 4 weeks, twice weekly for 4 weeks, then monthly; diazepam was used as required to control agitation. Eight patients completed the study period and they remained well throughout. Two continued beyond 6 months but relapsed at 8 and 9 months; no longer-term data were reported (Chanpattana, 1997). A second pilot followed a similar group for 12 months; it found that only 3 of 11 patients managed to remain well at 1 year after an acute ECT course (Chanpattana, 1998). In a controlled trial, 58 patients with medication-resistant schizophrenia, who had responded to acute treatment with bilateral ECT and flupenthixol, were randomised to three treatment groups: flupenthixol alone, cECT alone or a combination (Chanpattana et al, 1999b). Ratings were conducted by trained raters, who were blind to treatment group, using the BPRS. Forty-five patients completed the trial. Out of 15 patients in the single-treatment groups, 14 relapsed within 6 months compared with 6 of the 15 patients receiving flupenthixol plus cECT. Of the nine remaining responders in this group, therapeutic benefits were maintained during mECT treatment lasting from 3 to 17 months. This is the most rigorous trial to date and appears to indicate beneficial effects for maintenance ECT combined with a neuroleptic. Although encouraging, the samples used were small, and it is not clear whether other treatment possibil-ities, such as atypical neuroleptics (including clozapine), had been tried in these patients. A further, open, study by these workers, of cECT for patients with schizophrenia concurrently receiving flupenthixol, adds little to the debate (Chanpattana & Chakrabhand, 2001).

In summary, there is some evidence to suggest that, as in major depression, a few patients who respond to ECT treatment for schizophrenic symptoms may benefit from maintenance treatment. The characteristics of these patients, beyond initial response to ECT, are unclear, as are the optimal frequency and duration of treatment. Given that the efficacy of ECT for schizophrenia is unclear, however, considerable work in that area should be undertaken first to justify research into mECT. The American Psychiatric Association's Work Group on Schizophrenia concluded: 'The efficacy of maintenance ECT has not been studied adequately. However, it can be considered in the case of an ECT responder for whom pharmacological prophylaxis alone has been ineffective or cannot be tolerated' (American Psychiatric Association, 1997, p. 26).

Catatonia

The behavioural neurological syndrome of catatonia has been associated with schizophrenia since its inclusion as a subtype of dementia praecox by Kraepelin in 1896 and, later, of schizophrenia by Bleuler (Hawkins *et al*, 1995). This is a misconception and catatonia would perhaps better now be considered as a non-specific syndrome of multiple aetiologies. Its nosological status was in doubt during the drafting of DSM–IV but a move to create a separate diagnostic category did not prevail (Fink, 1994). Nevertheless, catatonic schizophrenia is well recognised, albeit rare. In one study, of 55 patients admitted with catatonic symptoms, only four satisfied the diagnostic criteria for schizophrenia (Abrams & Taylor, 1976), while a retrospective study found that, of 19 patients with diagnoses of catatonic schizophrenia on admission to hospital, only seven were classified as having schizophrenia on discharge, the rest being rediagnosed with affective or organic disorders (Pataki *et al*, 1992). The physical seriousness of catatonia – which can present as psychomotor disturbances leading to extreme behaviour such as hyperkinesis, stupor, catalepsy, negativism and anomalies of voluntary movement, which in turn are associated with dehydration, malnutrition, hyperpyrexia and outbursts of violence – merits urgent physical treatment. In such circumstances ECT has long been considered the treatment of choice. A recent alternative approach has been the use of benzodiazepines.

The only trial of ECT in catatonic schizophrenia of sufficient methodological rigour to be considered by the Cochrane review (Tharyan, 1996/2001) was that of Miller *et al* (1953), who studied ECT in patients with chronic catatonic schizophrenia and found no beneficial effects. Other literature comprises case reports of variable worth. Despite this, the American Psychiatric Association (1990) endorsed ECT as an effective treatment for the catatonic subtype of schizophrenia.

Hawkins *et al* (1995) reviewed all articles published over the 10 years from 1985 to 1994, selecting 70 of a total of 87 papers on the basis that they were written in English, reported clinical symptoms that met two or more DSM–IV diagnostic criteria for catatonia, detailed treatment interventions and responses, and neuroleptic malignant syndrome (NMS) was not suspected. The authors recorded 270 treatment episodes in 178 patients aged from 13 to 90 years, 52% of whom were male. The aetiologies were diverse, including medical and psychiatric causes, and no single cause predominated. The most common intervention (39%) was with benzodiazepines, mostly lorazepam. Seventy per cent of treatments with lorazepam alone resulted in a complete resolution of symptoms using a mean (s.d.) daily dose of 3.0 (2.8) mg. Other benzodiazepines (diazepam, clonazepam, midazolam, clorazepate, oxazepam) were used alone in 20 treatments, of which 16 produced complete resolution. ECT, used alone, comprised 20% of treatments, and it proved superior to benzodiazepines, in that it gave an 85% complete response rate. The authors reported that ECT 'demonstrated high efficacy' when used in combination with other treatments, although, in fact, the numbers are too small for such conclusions to be drawn with any confidence. Fifteen per cent ($n = 40$) of treatments were with antipsychotics alone, to which only 7.5% of patients responded completely. Moreover, four patients died, including two who had received neuroleptic treatment for catatonia; and four cases of NMS occurred in patients who had received antipsychotic treatment for their catatonia. There are many limitations to this work, beyond the reporting bias considered by the authors in their discussion. The failure to consider response to treatment within different aetiologies of catatonia limits the applicability of the findings to any one clinical syndrome, such as schizophrenia. At best, it is a review of case reports relating to a diverse syndrome of catatonia, without the methodological rigour of a clinical trial. Nevertheless, the authors conclude that catatonia (regardless of aetiology) should initially be treated with a benzodiazepine, proceeding to ECT if there is no improvement within 48–72 hours, if the patient's condition worsens, or if malignant catatonia (see below) is suspected.

In an attempt to relate the finding more clearly to schizophrenia, data were extracted from the paper by Hawkins *et al* (1995; their Table 1, pp. 350–359) where the patients studied had clear diagnoses of schizophrenia, catatonic schizophrenia or schizophreniform disorder. Nine studies were identified (Walter-Ryan, 1985; Salam *et al*, 1987; Rankel & Rankel, 1988; Ripley & Millson, 1988; Martényi *et al*, 1989; DeLisle, 1991; Mahmood, 1991; Smith & Lebegue, 1991; Van der Kelft *et al*, 1991 – for full references see Hawkins *et al*, 1995), which reported a total of 14 cases. Of these, 11 responded completely to benzodiazepine treatment, two following a failure of ECT and a variety of other treatments (Ripley & Millson, 1988; Smith & Lebegue, 1991). Only one showed a complete response to ECT, in combination with dantrolene following a failure of dantrolene alone (Van der Kelft *et al*, 1991) and one each responded to carbamazepine and bromocriptine.

A retrospective review of catatonic patients between 1985 and 1990 by Pataki *et al* (1992) found seven who satisfied DSM criteria for schizophrenia, of whom four were treated with ECT. One was reported to be 'much improved/recovered', while two were 'improved' and one unchanged. In a comparison group of seven patients with affective disorders, all five of the patients who were given ECT were 'much improved/recovered'. Although of interest, the picture is complicated by the variety of concurrent pharmacotherapies administered, including tricyclics, benzodiazepines and neuroleptics. The results are supported by those of Abrams (1997), who found that catatonic patients who fail to respond to ECT are more likely to have a primary diagnosis of schizophrenia, and by Escobar *et al* (2000), who showed a greater improvement among patients with catatonia associated with mood disorders than with schizophrenia.

Malignant (or 'lethal') catatonia

This is a variant of catatonia characterised by psychomotor abnormalities, delirium and hyperpyrexia, which, untreated, is rapidly fatal as a result of a combination of exhaustion and dehydration. The seminal review is that of Mann *et al* (1986), who identified 292 cases in the world literature from 1960, of which 117 were primarily schizophrenic. A further 71 cases were identified in a review of the literature from 1986 to 1992 (Singerman & Raheja, 1994), of which 50% had a diagnosis of schizophrenia. These articles indicate the seriousness of a condition with a mortality rate of 75–100% in the pre-neuroleptic era, 60% in the period 1960–85 and 31% between 1986 and 1992. The use of neuroleptics to treat the condition may be harmful, not least because of the difficulty of distinguishing the symptoms from those of NMS, into which it has been suggested it may develop (White & Robbins, 1991). There is some evidence, in the form of case reports, for the efficacy of ECT (see Krueger & Sackeim, 1995), which led Singerman & Raheja (1994) to recommend it as the first-line treatment once the diagnosis of malignant catatonia has been made. Other treatments, such as dantrolene or bromocriptine, may also be effective. One case report has been published since 1992, concerning a 47-year-old man with acute schizophrenia and malignant catatonia who could not be treated with neuroleptics as he had previously experienced NMS. No improvement was obtained with dantrolene, bromocriptine or lorazepam, but the condition was relieved by 11 applications of bilateral ECT (Boyarsky *et al*, 1999). No accounts were found of the use of atypical neuroleptics for malignant catatonia occurring in patients with schizophrenia. There is one account of a patient with a bipolar affective disorder whose malignant catatonic features responded to olanzapine at a dose of 30 mg/day (Cassidy *et al*, 2001).

Summary

Studies of ECT for the treatment of catatonia are confined largely to single case reports, although there are also a few small series. Most studies consider catatonia as a clinical syndrome in its own right and fail to examine the differential response of different underlying conditions such as schizophrenia, or affective or organic disorders. When these factors are taken into consideration, the evidence for the beneficial effect of ECT in catatonic schizophrenia would appear to be less than that in affective disorders. Benzodiazepines and barbiturates have also been found to be effective, and it seems that benzodiazepines offer a safe alternative to ECT, and one that is less invasive. Indeed, the absence of randomised clinical trials, particularly studies of sham ECT versus true ECT in catatonic schizophrenia, has led one author to suggest that the barbiturate anaesthetic induction agent may be the effective element in ECT for catatonia (DeLisle, 1992). There is clearly a need for more research, but, on the basis of the available evidence, the first-line treatment should be benzodiazepines, before proceeding to ECT, in uncomplicated cases of catatonia. For malignant catatonia, or in circumstances where use of benzodiazepines is contraindicated, ECT should be the first-line treatment. Conventional neuroleptics may be harmful: their use is cautioned, and contraindicated in malignant catatonia.

Schizoaffective disorder

Little recent attention has been paid to schizoaffective disorder, despite observations that the presence of affective symptoms in schizophrenia may predict a good response to ECT (World Health Organization, 1979). No conclusions could be drawn by the Cochrane review since only one study containing schizoaffective patients met the criteria for inclusion and these subjects were in any case excluded as they could not be separated from a heterogeneous group of patients with affective disorders (Tharyan, 1996/2001). Only one study has looked exclusively at the response of schizoaffective disorders to ECT, and it reported a strong response in nine patients who had failed to respond to two different antipsychotic medications (Ries *et al*, 1981). Nevertheless, there are a number of case reports of a favourable response on the part of patients with a depressed type of schizoaffective disorder, who have been said to respond as well as patients with psychotic depression (Lapensée, 1992).

Schizoaffective disorder is a heterogeneous condition of uncertain nosological affiliation and there is little clarity in the research as to which symptoms respond to ECT. It is unclear whether the affective and schizophrenic symptoms are equally responsive or whether manic and depressive subtypes respond similarly. Indeed, it is possible that the improvement seen in case reports represents a short-term relief of affective symptoms alone and that the schizoaffective disorder, per se, is relatively unchanged. Much research is needed and the most that can be concluded at present is that ECT may provide relief for some symptoms of some patients with schizoaffective disorder.

Schizophreniform disorder

Schizophrenic symptoms of brief onset associated with good social functioning are included as a separate category of DSM–IV (American Psychiatric Association, 1994) but not ICD–10 (World Health Organization, 1992). Although it has been included as a purist diagnosis in some studies of acute schizophrenia, neither the Cochrane review nor the current literature search found studies that looked specifically at this group. Given the evidence above for acute schizophrenia, there is no indication for the use of ECT in this disorder.

Delusional disorder

Although delusional disorder is probably unrelated, nosologically, to schizophrenia (Fear *et al*, 1998), it is convenient to consider the few case reports of ECT in delusional disorder in this chapter. Fink (1995) suggested that ECT was an 'antidelusional agent', given its reported efficacy for a variety of conditions in which delusions feature as a symptom. The supporting evidence consists of only two reports of delusional infestation (Hopkinson, 1973; Bebbington, 1976) and one reporting erotomanic delusions (Remington & Jeffries, 1994). It is likely that response in these cases was attributable to an improvement of underlying mood disorders.

Technique

Most of the research into the effect of electrode placement on efficacy in schizophrenia was conducted more than 30 years ago and is of uncertain relevance to contemporary practice; substantial, but unexplained, discontinuation of treatment was another method-ological problem that complicates interpretation of the findings (see Sackeim, 2003). There is preliminary evidence that the extent to which the electrical dose exceeds the seizure threshold is correlated with the rate of improvement, but not final efficacy, in patients with schizophrenia who respond to bilateral ECT (Sackeim, 2003).

Many contradictory assertions have been made concerning the frequency of treatments and length of course, some authors suggesting courses of 20 treatments or more (e.g. Fink, 1979). In fact, there is no good evidence to support these views and more recent studies have tended towards an identical approach to that used in treating depression, with a course of 6–12 treatments.

Adverse effects

There is no evidence of particular adverse effects being more common in patients with schizophrenia than those, say, with depression who are given ECT.

Discussion

Schizophrenia was one of the first indications given for ECT and, since 1938, a vast literature has explored many aspects of its use. Sadly, the majority of these publications consist of case reports and anecdotes, so that there is a dearth of good-quality clinical trials based upon sound methods. Most of the work on ECT as the sole intervention dates from before neuroleptics were widely available, and although there is some evidence to support its efficacy for patients with acute schizophrenia, antipsychotic drugs appear to be superior. The studies upon which this view is based relate only to typical neuroleptics and it is likely that, given the variety of atypicals now available, the advantage of pharmacotherapy over ECT will be assured. There is currently no research to support this, however, and in countries with more limited therapeutic options ECT is likely to remain an important intervention (Agarwal *et al*, 1992; Daradkeh *et al*, 1998; Tang & Ungvari, 2001). There is no evidence to suggest that the beneficial effects of ECT persist beyond the short term.

Recent attention has turned towards adding ECT to neuroleptic treatment in patients who have failed to respond fully to neuroleptics. There are no good-quality studies to support this approach, but neither is there any information to suggest that the combination of ECT with neuroleptics, including clozapine, is intrinsically harmful. Approximately a third of patients with schizophrenia have symptoms that are resistant to all neuroleptics, including clozapine (Meltzer, 1995), and in this group a trial of ECT is an option and relatively safe. There is a need for good-quality research in this area. Even if effective, ECT appears to offer only short-term relief of symptoms and there is some evidence to support the use of maintenance ECT as an adjunct to neuroleptics for prophylaxis in this group.

It is impossible to examine the evidence on the effect ECT on catatonic schizophrenia in isolation from other causes of catatonia. No clinical trials have been conducted but evidence from case studies suggests that benzodiazepines, particularly lorazepam, provide a safe alternative which is at least as effective as ECT in alleviating acute symptoms. Neuroleptics appear ineffective and may be harmful in malignant catatonia, which is often indistinguishable from NMS. It is recommended that, unless contraindicated, a trial of benzodiazepines is undertaken for up to 72 hours, before proceeding to ECT in the event of a partial response or non-response. For malignant catatonia, ECT is the treatment of choice.

There is some evidence to support the relief of affective symptoms in schizoaffective disorder and ECT is a therapeutic option when pharmacological interventions have failed. In the case of severe depressive or manic symptoms, it is recommended that treatment accords with the recommendations applying to major depression and hypomania (see Chapter 2). ECT is not indicated in schizophreniform psychosis. In delusional disorder it may be effective as a treatment of last resort, but evidence is scanty and it is probably most effective where affective symptoms are present.

No recommendations can be made with regard to technique and a standard bilateral electrode placement and twice-weekly applications given as clinically indicated offer the best results. There are no particular problems or adverse effects specific to ECT in schizophrenia.

Recommendations

Schizophrenia

The treatment of choice for acute schizophrenia is antipsychotic drug treatment. ECT may be considered as an option for treatment-resistant schizophrenia, where treatment with clozapine has already proven ineffective or intolerable. There is presently no evidence to support the use of ECT as a maintenance treatment in schizophrenia.

Catatonia

Catatonia is a syndrome that may complicate several psychiatric and medical conditions. ECT may be considered as a first-line treatment in life-threatening malignant catatonia. In less severe cases, the treatment of choice is a benzodiazepine drug; most experience is with lorazepam. ECT may be indicated when treatment with lorazepam has been ineffective.

Acknowledgements

The author would like to thank Bill Evans of the Gloucestershire Partnership Trust library service and Alex Celini, research assistant at the Royal College of Psychiatrists, for their assistance with this paper.

References

Abrams, R. (1997) Technique of electro-convulsive therapy: theory. In *Electroconvulsive Therapy* (ed. R. Abrams), pp. 185–189. New York: Oxford University Press.

Abrams, R. & Taylor, M. A. (1976) Catatonia. A prospective clinical study. *Archives of General Psychiatry*, **33**, 579–581.

Agarwal, A. K., Andrade, C. & Reddy, M. C. (1992) The practice of ECT in India: issues relating to the administration of ECT. *Indian Journal of Psychiatry*, **34**, 285–297.

American Psychiatric Association (1994) *Diagnostic and Statistical Manual of Mental Disorders* (4th edn) (DSM–IV). Washington, DC: APA.

American Psychiatric Association (1997) *Practice Guidelines for the Treatment of Patients with Schizophrenia.* Washington, DC: APA.

American Psychiatric Association Task Force on ECT (1990) *The Practice of ECT: Recommendations for Treatment, Training and Priviledging.* Washington, DC: APA.

Barnes, T. R. E., McEvedy, C. J. B. & Nelson, H. E. (1996) Management of treatment resistant schizophrenia unresponsive to clozapine. *British Journal of Psychiatry*, **169** (suppl. 31), 31–40.

Bebbington, P. E. (1976) Monosymptomatic hypochondriasis, abnormal illness behaviour and suicide. *British Journal of Psychiatry*, **128**, 475–478.

Benatov, R., Sirota, P. & Megged, S. (1996) Neuroleptic-resistant schizophrenia treated with clozapine and ECT. *Convulsive Therapy*, **12**, 117–121.

Bhatia, S. C., Bhatia, S. K. & Gupta, S. (1998) Concurrent administration of clozapine and ECT: a successful treatment strategy for a patient with treatment-resistant schizophrenia. *Journal of ECT*, **14**, 280–283.

Boyarsky, B. K., Fuller, M., Early, T., *et al* (1999) Malignant catatonia-induced respiratory failure with response to ECT. *Journal of ECT*, **15**, 232–236.

Cassidy, E. M., O'Brien, M., Osman, M. F., *et al* (2001) Lethal catatonia responding to high-dose olanzapine therapy. *Journal of Psychopharmacology*, **15**, 302–304.

Chanpattana, W. (1997) Continuation electroconvulsive therapy in schizophrenia: a pilot study. *Journal of the Medical Association of Thailand*, **80**, 311–318.

Chanpattana, W. (1998) Maintenance ECT in schizophrenia: a pilot study. *Journal of the Medical Association of Thailand*, **81**, 17–24.

Chanpattana, W. (2000) Maintenance ECT in treatment-resistant schizophrenia. *Journal of the Medical Association of Thailand*, **83**, 657–662.

Chanpattana, W. & Chakrabhand, M. L. S. (2001) Factors influencing treatment frequency of ECT in schizophrenia. *Journal of ECT*, **17**, 190–194.

Chanpattana, W., Chakrabhand, M. L. S., Kongsakon, R., *et al* (1999a) Short-term effect of combined ECT and neuroleptic therapy in treatment-resistant schizophrenia. *Journal of ECT*, **15**, 129–139.

Chanpattana, W., Chakrabhand, M. L., Sackeim, H. A., *et al* (1999b) Continuation ECT in treatment-resistant schizophrenia: a controlled study. *Journal of ECT*, **15**, 178–192.

Christison, G. W., Kirch, D. G. & Wyatt, R. J. (1991) When symptoms persist: choosing among alternative somatic treatments for schizophrenia. *Schizophrenia Bulletin*, **17**, 217–245.

Daradkeh, T. K., Saad, A. & Younis, Y. (1998) Contemporary status of electroconvulsive therapy in a teaching psychiatric unit in the United Arab Emirates. *Nordisk Psykiatrisk Tidsskrift*, **52**, 481–485.

DeLisle, J. D. (1992) Reply to SJ Masiar; M Fink: Failure to use ECT in treatment of catatonia (letter). *American Journal of Psychiatry*, **149**, 145–146.

Escobar, R., Rios, A., Montoya, I. D., *et al* (2000) Clinical and cerebral blood flow changes in catatonic patients treated with ECT. *Journal of Psychosomatic Research*, **49**, 423–429.

Fear, C. F., McMonagle, T. & Healy, D. (1998) Delusional disorder: boundaries of a syndrome. *European Psychiatry*, **13**, 210–218.

Fink, M. (1979) *Convulsive Therapy: Theory and Practice*. New York: Raven Press.

Fink, M. (1994) Catatonia in DSM–IV. *Biological Psychiatry*, **36**, 431–433.

Fink, M. (1995) Electroconvulsive therapy in delusional disorders. *Psychiatric Clinics of North America*, **18**, 393–406.

Fink, M. (1998) ECT and clozapine in schizophrenia. *Journal of ECT*, **14**, 223–226.

Fink, M. (2001) Convulsive therapy: a review of the first 55 years. *Journal of Affective Disorders*, **63**, 1–15.

Fink, M. & Sackeim H. A. (1996) Convulsive therapy in schizophrenia? *Schizophrenia Bulletin*, **22**, 27–39.

Hawkins, J. M., Archer, K. J., Strakowski, S. M., *et al* (1995) Somatic treatment of catatonia. *International Journal of Psychiatry in Medicine*, **25**, 345–369.

Hirose, S., Ashby, C. R., Jr & Mills, M. J. (2001) The effectiveness of ECT combined with risperidone against aggression in schizophrenia. *Journal of ECT*, **17**, 22–26.

Hopkinson, G. (1973) The psychiatric syndrome of infestation. *Psychiatric Clinics of North America*, **6**, 330–345.

James, D. V. & Gray, N. S. (1999) Elective combined electroconvulsive and clozaril therapy. *International Clinical Psychopharmacology*, **14**, 69–72.

Johns, C. A. & Thompson, J. W. (1995) Adjunctive treatments in schizophrenia: pharmacotherapies and electroconvulsive therapy. *Schizophrenia Bulletin*, **21**, 607–619.

Kales, H. C., Dequardo, J. R. & Tandon, R. (1999) Combined electroconvulsive therapy and clozapine in treatment-resistant schizophrenia. *Progress in Neuropsychopharmacology and Biological Psychiatry*, **23**, 547–556.

Karliner, W. & Wehrheim, H. (1965) Maintenance convulsive treatments. *American Journal of Psychiatry*, **121**, 1113–1115.

Klapheke, M. M. (1993) Combining ECT and antipsychotic agents: benefits and risks. *Convulsive Therapy*, **9**, 241–255.

Kramer, B. A. (1999) A naturalistic review of maintenance ECT at a university setting. *Journal of ECT*, **15**, 262–269.

Krueger, R. B. & Sackeim, H. A. (1995) Electroconvulsive therapy and schizophrenia. In *Schizophrenia* (eds S. R. Hirsch & D. R. Weinberger), pp. 503–545. Oxford: Blackwell.

Kupchik, M., Spivak, B., Mester, R., *et al* (2000) Combined electroconvulsive–clozapine therapy. *Clinical Neuropharmacology*, **23**, 14–16.

Lapensée, M. A. (1992) A review of schizoaffective disorder: II. Somatic treatment. *Canadian Journal of Psychiatry*, **37**, 347–349.

Lehman, A. F., Steinwachs, D. M., Dixon, L. B., *et al* (1998) Translating research into practice: the Schizophrenia Patient Outcomes Research Team (PORT) treatment recommendations. *Schizophrenia Bulletin*, **24**, 1–10.

Mann, S. C., Caroff, S. N., Bleier, H. R., *et al* (1986) Lethal catatonia. *American Journal of Psychiatry*, **143**, 1374–1381.

Masiar, S. J. & Johns, C. A. (1991) ECT following clozapine (letter). *British Journal of Psychiatry*, **158**, 135–136.

Meltzer, H. Y. (1995) Atypical antipsychotic drug therapy for treatment-resistant schizophrenia. In *Schizophrenia* (eds S. R. Hirsch & D. R. Weinberger), pp. 485–502. Oxford: Blackwell.

Miller, D. H., Clancy, J. & Cumming, E. (1953) A comparison between undirectional current nonconvulsive electrical stimulation given with Reiters machine, standard alternating current electroshock (Cerletti method), and Pentothal in chronic schizophrenia. *American Journal of Psychiatry*, **109**, 617–620.

Pataki, J., Zervas, I. M. & Jandorf, L. (1992) Catatonia in a university inpatient service (1985–1990). *Convulsive Therapy*, **8**, 163–173.

Remington, G. J. & Jeffries, J. J. (1994) Erotomanic delusions and electroconvulsive therapy: a case series. *Journal of Clinical Psychiatry*, **55**, 306–308.

Ries, R. K., Wilson, L., Bokan, J. A., *et al* (1981) ECT in medication resistant schizoaffective disorder. *Comprehensive Psychiatry*, **22**, 167–173.

Sackeim, H. A. (2003) Electroconvulsive therapy and schizophrenia. In *Schizophrenia* (eds S. R. Hirsch & D. R. Weinberger) (2nd edn), pp. 517–551. Edinburgh: Blackwell.

Sackeim, H. A., Prudic, J., Devanand, D. P., *et al* (1990) The impact of medication resistance and continuation pharmacotherapy on relapse following response to electroconvulsive therapy in major depression. *Journal of Clinical Psychopharmacology*, **10**, 96–104.

Sarita, E. P., Janakiramaiah, N., Gangadhar, B. N., *et al* (1998) Efficacy of combined ECT after two weeks of neuroleptics in schizophrenia: a double blind controlled study. *National Institute of Mental Health and Neurosciences Journal*, **16**, 243–251.

Singerman, B. & Raheja, R. (1994) Malignant catatonia – a continuing reality. *Annals of Clinical Psychiatry*, **6**, 259–66.

Stiebel, V. G. (1995) Maintenance electroconvulsive therapy for chronic mentally ill patients: a case series. *Psychiatric Services*, **46**, 265–268.

Tang, K.-W. & Ungvari, G. S. (2001) Electroconvulsive therapy in rehabilitation: the Hong Kong experience. *Psychiatric Services*, **52**, 303–306.

Tharyan, P. (1996/2001) Electroconvulsive therapy for schizophrenia (Cochrane review). In *The Cochrane Library, Issue 4*. Oxford: Update Software.

White, D. A. C. & Robbins, A. H. (1991) Catatonia: harbinger of the neuroleptic syndrome. *British Journal of Psychiatry*, **158**, 419–421.

World Health Organization (1979) *Schizophrenia: An International Follow-Up Study*. New York: Wiley.

World Health Organization (1992) *International Classification of Diseases* (10th revision) (ICD–10). New York: Wiley.

CHAPTER 5

The use of ECT in neuropsychiatric disorders

Michael R. Trimble and Ennapadam S. Krishnamoorthy

Electroconvulsive therapy has come a long way from von Meduna's early theory of antagonism between epilepsy and schizophrenia to its application today in a range of neuropsychiatric disorders. Meduna (1935) postulated that epilepsy and psychosis were antagonistic, and that seizures therefore could be used to treat schizophrenia. While this idea is in the broad sense no longer the basis for the use of ECT per se, the antagonism between seizures and behavioural disorder, also seen in another clinical setting, the so-called 'forced normalisation and alternative psychosis' of epilepsy (Krishnamoorthy & Trimble, 1999), is but one example of antagonisms in clinical neuropsychiatry. Other examples include: the creation of brain lesions to treat psychiatric conditions such as depression and obsessive–compulsive disorders (psychosurgery); the treatment of schizophrenia with neuroleptics, leading in turn to convulsions; the treatment of parkinsonism with L-dopa, leading to improvement in the symptoms of that disease but also psychotic symptoms; and temporal lobectomy for patients with epilepsy, producing seizure freedom but also associated with psychiatric disorders such as depression and psychosis (Trimble, 1996).

Rooted in such a background of biological antagonism one would expect ECT to have established itself, or alternatively been eliminated, as a form of treatment in neurology and neuropsychiatry. In this review we examine the objective evidence for the use of ECT in neurological and neuropsychiatric disorders.

Parkinson's disease

Parkinson's disease (PD) is a neurodegenerative disorder characterised by akinesia, tremor, rigidity, postural instability and disturbances in mood and cognition. Its medical management is complicated by the 'on–off' syndrome (abrupt changes in motor function ranging from excessive dyskinetic movements to freezing instability) and debilitating (often drug-induced) psychotic symptoms, such as delusions and hallucinations (Kellner & Bernstein, 1993). Electroconvulsive therapy is known to enhance dopaminergic function in both animals and humans. The role of ECT, therefore, as a safe and effective modality of treatment for PD, without some of the aforementioned side-effects, indeed with improvement in some of the behavioural features, has been the source of considerable debate.

Comprehensive reviews have looked at the efficacy of ECT as a modality of treatment in PD. Faber & Trimble (1991) concluded their review of the early literature and all 27 modern reports published by then as follows: 'approximately half of patients with severe PD might be expected to have a meaningful response of sufficient duration to make ECT a worthwhile adjunctive consideration when current therapies are unsatisfactory, especially if maintenance ECT can be continued when warranted'. Other reviewers, for example Kellner & Bernstein (1993) and Krystal & Coffey (1997), have also concluded that ECT is a safe adjunctive treatment for both motor and affective symptoms in patients with PD who do not respond well to drugs. It has been pointed out that future research must focus on optimal ECT techniques in PD.

Reviewing the literature, the overwhelming number of single and multiple case reports contrast with the paucity of well-designed clinical trials. Interestingly, however, the vast majority of these case reports have shown positive results, with very few studies failing to demonstrate a response to ECT among patients with PD.

Following on from earlier prospective research examining patients with the on–off syndrome (Balldin et al, 1980, 1981), Andersen et al (1987) conducted a double-blind trial of ECT in 11 patients with PD. The patients were aged between 51 and 81 years, suffered from the on–off syndrome, and were described as being non-depressed and non-dementing. Patients were randomly allocated to either active ECT or 'sham' ECT. The patients given active ECT had significantly ($P<0.05$) longer 'on' phases after ECT than did the sham ECT group. We could find no other controlled trials in a detailed review of several standard databases.

A prospective clinical trial of bilateral ECT in PD, in seven patients, carried out by Douyon et al (1989), also showed very positive results. Mean (s.d.) scores on the New York University Parkinson's Disease Scale fell from 65 (15) to 32 (6), with all five sub-scales showing a roughly equal response.

Moellentine et al (1998), in a retrospective study of 25 patients with PD matched for age and sex with 25 patients receiving ECT for psychiatric symptoms, found ECT to improve psychiatric symptoms in both groups, as expected, but also, at least transiently, motor symptoms, in 14 of 25 subjects in the PD group.

Pridmore & Pollard (1996) studied 14 patients with PD but without comorbid psychiatric illness, who were given ECT for motor symptoms and followed up over 30 months (though data were incomplete for two patients). About a third had either no benefit or mild benefit that lasted 2 weeks or less, a third had mild benefit that lasted from 4 weeks to 30 months, and a third had marked benefit that lasted from 10 weeks to 35 months.

Thus there is some evidence that suggests a role for ECT as an adjunctive treatment for the motor symptoms of PD. In addition, ECT can be given safely for comorbid affective disorder in these patients, if clinically warranted. Several reviewers have examined issues such as electrode placement, type of ECT, frequency, dosing, continuation of L-dopa and other PD drugs, and duration of response. There is little evidence that would help one make firm recommendations. It has been opined, however, that continuous and maintenance therapy with ambulatory ECT will allow improvement to be maintained in both motor disorder and mood disorder (Krystal & Coffey, 1997).

Kellner & Bernstein (1993), following on from Zervas & Fink (1991), and Rasmussen & Abrams (1991) have made certain recommendations for clinicians about the use of ECT for the movement disorder in PD. These remain relevant and are summarised below:

- Include only patients refractory to drug treatment of PD, usually those with severe disability.
- Gain patients' informed consent, and emphasise the limited putative benefit and rapid relapse.
- Reduce the dose of L-dopa by half, and discontinue adjunctive treatment to prevent emergent dyskinesias and post-ECT delirium.
- Brief-pulse unilateral ECT is to be preferred, at least to begin with, as it has been shown to be effective in reports and gives fewer cognitive side-effects; there is the possibility of a switch to bilateral electrode placement after three treatments if there is no response.
- Give a substantial supra-threshold electrical dosage (75% of the device's maximum dose).
- Aim to induce generalised tonic–clonic convulsive activity, as would be done when giving ECT for psychiatric disorders.
- Stop the treatment as soon as maximum benefit is attained (i.e. until no further benefit is seen after each of two consecutive treatments). Improvement (if any) almost always starts after the third treatment. Cease the administration of ECT if no improvement occurs after the sixth bilateral treatment.
- Reinstate optimal PD medication as soon as ECT is terminated, and return L-dopa dosages to previous levels (assuming there are no intolerance adverse effects) and restart the patient on any previously helpful adjunctive agents.

- Consider the use of intermittent single out-patient ECT sessions ('maintenance' ECT), to prevent or delay the return of extra-pyramidal symptoms, using a trial and error approach of pro-gressively increasing the inter-treatment interval from, for example, once a week initially, to the longest interval that will sustain improvement effectively (e.g. monthly).

It is important to recognise that these recommendations are limited in that they are derived from clinical experience of ECT, in a number of patients with PD, rather than from well-designed clinical trials. However, in the absence of hard evidence, there is an acknowledged role for such expert recommendations. It is also important to recognise that these recommendations should be considered alongside other general recommendations for ECT, outlined elsewhere in the present book, as well as sound clinical judgement in each individual case. Importantly, these recommendations are given in a format that might lend itself to empirical testing in the future.

Other movement disorders in neuropsychiatry

The use of ECT in many other movement disorders has been the subject of case reports and some reviews, although there have been no controlled clinical trials of note.

It has been used with some success in neuroleptic-induced parkin-sonism, where it has been reported to improve the motor aspects of that condition quite significantly (Gangadhar et al, 1983; Goswami et al, 1989).

Neuroleptic malignant syndrome (NMS) can follow exposure to neuroleptic drugs and is attributed to abnormal dopaminergic activity in the brain. It constitutes a medical emergency, as it has considerable morbidity and mortality, even in the best settings. It has been suggested that NMS can be treated effectively with ECT. Indeed, in a review of 48 reported cases of NMS treated with ECT, Davis et al (1991) found that patients receiving no specific treatment had a higher mortality rate (21%) than those receiving ECT (10.3%) or pharmacotherapy. However, no controlled trials of ECT in NMS have been carried out, and concerns about the safety of succinyl choline in NMS have been raised, as the drug has the potential to cause malignant hyperthermia, a condition with manifestations akin to NMS, but with possibly a different patho-physiology.

There is considerable literature on the use of ECT in tardive dyskinesia (TD), much of it surprisingly contradictory and inconclusive: several case reports suggest that ECT improves this condition, while several others report that TD worsens with ECT (Faber & Trimble, 1991; Krystal & Coffey, 1997). Similarly contradictory reports and the absence of clinical trials characterise the literature relating to ECT and other neuroleptic-induced movement disorders, such as tardive dystonia, and also conditions like Gilles de la Tourette syndrome and other tic disorders (see Faber & Trimble, 1991, for a review). The reason for such variability in response in TD and allied disorders may be the heterogeneous nature of these disorders. Other conditions in which the utility of ECT is unclear include Huntingdon's disease and progressive supranuclear palsy (PSP). In general, however, there is no suggestion that ECT is unsafe in these disorders, with the caveat that emergent paradoxical movements have been observed in some subjects (Flaherty et al, 1984). Further, the patient should be counselled about the inconclusive nature of the evidence for efficacy.

Other disorders at the interface between neurology and psychiatry

Catatonia is a syndrome associated with a variety of medical and neurological conditions, including diffuse brain injury, status epilepticus, thyroid and parathyroid disorders, encephalopathy (metabolic and infectious) and so on. The psychiatric causes of catatonia include affective disorders, schizophrenia and even hysteria, and in this context it is important to remember that catatonia is a clinical syndrome caused more often by medical disorders, rather than an independent disease entity (Gelenberg, 1976). The evidence for the efficacy of ECT in catatonia is reviewed in Chapter 4. When considering the cost–benefit analysis of the use of ECT in catatonia it is important to remember the cautionary note of Krystal & Coffey (1997); they pointed out that, 'when administering ECT to such patients, it is important to carry out a careful evaluation of the aetiology of the catatonia in order to determine whether the underlying process increases the risks of ECT'.

While the use of ECT is known to lead to the development of short-term cognitive impairment, it has become clear that ECT may have a role to play in the management of dementia. Comorbid depression is a prominent feature of dementia, with a quarter to three-quarters of subjects with dementia affected, depending on the type of dementia and the type of rating of depressive symptoms and syndromes. There is little evidence to suggest that ECT may worsen dementia in the long term, and a number of case reports support the use of ECT in the treatment of dementia with depression. Price & McAllister (1989) reviewed the cases of 56 patients with both dementia (Alzheimer's disease, multi-infarct dementia, Parkinson's disease and so on) and depression who were treated with ECT. They found an overall depression response rate of 73%. Further, nearly one-third of this sample had an improvement in condition, although a number experienced delirium during the course of treatment.

As the differential diagnosis of dementia and depression is complicated, because subjects are often unable to report classic symptoms of depression such as anhedonia, there is much to be said in favour of a therapeutic trial of ECT for patients who suffer from dementia and depression in tandem (see Kellner & Bernstein, 1993, for review). It is worth noting that some have recommended unilateral non-dominant ECT rather than bilateral ECT in the presence of cognitive blunting, with a view to decreasing post-seizure confusion.

Post-stroke depression is a frequent and disabling condition that is considered to be a direct consequence of brain injury. In a review of the records of 193 patients with stroke and depression, treated at the Massachusetts General Hospital, Murray et al (1986) found 14 to have had ECT, 12 of whom showed improvement, and none showed deterioration. Interestingly, cognition was found to improve in five out of six patients with 'cognitive impairment'. Coffey et al (1989) have reported that older patients with white-matter lesions (hyperintensity) on magnetic resonance scans showed an excellent response to ECT. That these white-matter hyperintensity lesions have been attributed to vascular disease is of interest.

It is common experience that repeated ECT administration leads to an increase in seizure threshold, with progressive treatments requiring larger doses. Animal studies show that electroconvulsive seizures (ECS) have anticonvulsant properties in that they raise seizure threshold and block kindling. The elegant work of Sackeim et al (1987a,b) on the effects of ECT on seizure threshold has led to an understanding of the potent anticonvulsant properties of ECT. Sackeim et al (1983) have also demonstrated a reduction in cerebral flow after ECT, using the xenon-inhalation technique, and postulated that the neural hypometabolic state and anticonvulsant effect may be due to the effects of ECT on gamma-aminobutyric acid (GABA).

Probably the only clinical study of the anticonvulsant effects of ECT has been in children. Two children with intractable epilepsy were treated with ECT for seizure control. One child showed a change in seizure pattern with treatment, which at greater intensity was also effective in stopping non-convulsive status epilepticus. The other child showed a decrease in spontaneous seizure frequency during short-term treatment. These findings suggest a role for ECT in the management of intractable epilepsy in children who are not candidates for epileptic surgery (Griesemer et al, 1997). It has been argued that ECT, a relatively benign and non-invasive treatment, may be preferred to radical methods such as epilepsy surgery (Kellner & Bernstein, 1993), but there have been no controlled trials of ECT in refractory epilepsy.

While the presence of a space-occupying cerebral lesion, and raised intracranial tension due to this and any other cause, are conventionally considered to be contraindications for ECT, there are a number of case reports that suggest the relative safety and utility of ECT in patients with cerebral tumours and comorbid psychopathology, even following craniotomy (see Starkstein & Migliorelli, 1993, for example). Maltbie *et al* (1980) pooled data from seven retrospective studies of 28 cases reported in the literature. While results indicated a high morbidity and even mortality, the authors pointed out that a number of patients in this series had undiagnosed brain tumours. Twenty-one per cent of the series of patients did show a good behavioural response to ECT, without complications. It has been suggested that in patients with small lesions, without oedema or signs of raised intracranial pressure, ECT may be used following a careful risk–benefit analysis, including neurosurgical consultation, as the use of steroids, antihypertensive agents and hyperventilation may diminish the rise in intracranial pressure (Weiner & Coffey, 1993).

Electroconvulsive therapy has also been used successfully in delirium due to a number of conditions. It has been argued that it is effective for the treatment of neuropsychiatric symptoms of delirium, and should be considered when other treatments fail (Krystal & Coffey, 1997). It must be noted, however, that ECT is known to cause delirium in a number of subjects, particularly those with lesions of the basal ganglia (Figiel *et al*, 1990), and caution therefore needs to be exercised in adopting it as a treatment for refractory delirium, particularly in the absence of clinical trials.

It has also been used with varying effects in patients with a number of other neurological disorders and comorbid neuropsychiatric conditions, including cerebral aneurysm, multiple sclerosis, cerebral lupus, neurosyphilis, traumatic brain injury, brain infections, myasthenia gravis and muscular dystrophy (for reviews see Kellner & Bernstein, 1993; Krystal & Coffey, 1997). The vast majority of these are individual case reports, and no significant adverse effects have been consistently reported.

Discussion

It is evident from this review that while ECT has been used extensively in a number of neurological and neuropsychiatric disorders, there is little by way of empirical evidence to recommend its routine use in these conditions. The one disorder in which ECT has been used successfully to ameliorate both neurological (motor) and neuropsychiatric (affective and psychotic) symptoms is PD. It is also the only disorder in this group in which some clinical trials have been performed, including a double-blind controlled study (Andersen *et al*, 1987). While a number of issues with regard to the use of ECT in PD remain unresolved, it seems fair to conclude that it can be used safely for the treatment of PD, provided the recommendations made here are followed.

The only other neuropsychiatric disorder in which ECT has been shown to be consistently helpful is catatonia. In this condition, however, the evidence has largely been drawn from case series and individual case reports, and prospective clinical trials are indicated. There are other conditions, such as dementia with depression and post-stroke depression, where case series and individual reports seem to indicate that ECT is relatively safe and efficacious, provided it is used judiciously.

Then there are disorders such as the neuroleptic-induced movement disorders, such as drug-induced parkinsonism, tardive dyskinesia and dystonia, where ECT may be tried with relative safety, although there is no hard evidence for its use.

Finally, there are disorders such as cerebral tumours with comorbid psychopathology, epilepsy, and NMS, where a trial of ECT may lead to beneficial effects, provided a great deal of caution is exercised and a careful risk analysis undertaken in each case.

Recommendations

- Electroconvulsive therapy is a safe, adjunctive treatment for both motor and affective symptoms in sufferers of PD with severe disability despite medical treatment.
- Catatonia is a syndrome that may complicate several psychiatric and medical conditions. The treatment of choice is a benzo-diazepine drug; most experience is with lorazepam. ECT may be indicated when treatment with lorazepam has been ineffective.
- The use of ECT remains an experimental treatment for neuro-psychiatric disorders such as neuroleptic malignant syndrome, Huntingdon's disease and treatment-resistant epilepsy.

References

Andersen, K., Balldin, J., Gottfries, C. G., *et al* (1987) A double-blind evaluation of electroconvulsive therapy in Parkinson's disease with 'on–off' phenomena. *Acta Neurologica Scandinavica*, **76**, 191–199.

Balldin, J., Eden, S., Granerus, A. K., *et al* (1980) Electroconvulsive therapy in Parkinson's syndrome with 'on–off' phenomenon. *Journal of Neural Transmission*, **47**, 11–21.

Balldin, J., Granerus, A. K., Lindstedt, G., *et al* (1981) Predictors for improvement after electroconvulsive therapy in parkinsonian patients with 'on–off' symptoms. *Journal of Neural Transmission*, **52**, 199–211.

Coffey, C. E., Figiel, G. S., Djang, W. T., et al (1989) White matter hyperintensity on magnetic resonance imaging: clinical and neuroanatomic correlates in the depressed elderly. *Journal of Neuropsychiatry*, **1**, 135–144.

Davis, J., Janicak, P., Sakkas, P., et al (1991) Electroconvulsive therapy in the treatment of the neuroleptic malignant syndrome. *Convulsive Therapy*, **7**, 111–120.

Douyon, R., Serby, M., Klutchko, B., et al (1989) ECT and Parkinson's disease revisited: a 'naturalistic' study. *American Journal of Psychiatry*, **146**, 1451–1455.

Faber, R. & Trimble, M. R. (1991) Electroconvulsive therapy in Parkinson's disease and other movement disorders. *Movement Disorders*, **6**, 293–303.

Figiel, G. S., Coffey, C. E., Djang, W. T., et al (1990) Brain magnetic resonance imaging findings in ECT-induced delirium. *Journal of Neuropsychiatry and Clinical Neurosciences*, **2**, 53–58.

Flaherty, J. A., Naidu, J. & Dysken, M. (1984) ECT, emergent dyskinesia, and depression. *American Journal of Psychiatry*, **141**, 803–809.

Gangadhar, B. N., Roychowdhury, J. & Channabasavanna, S. M. (1983) ECT and drug-induced parkinsonism. *Indian Journal of Psychiatry*, **25**, 212–213.

Gelenberg, A. (1976) The catatonic syndrome. *Lancet*, **i**, 1339–1341.

Goswami, U., Dutta, S., Kuruvilla, K., et al (1989) Electroconvulsive therapy in neuroleptic-induced parkinsonism. *Biological Psychiatry*, **26**, 234–238.

Griesemer, D. A., Kellner, C. H., Beale, M. D., et al (1997) Electroconvulsive therapy for the treatment of intractable seizures. Initial findings in two children. *Neurology*, **49**, 1389–1392.

Kellner, C. H. & Bernstein, H. J. (1993) ECT as a treatment for neurologic illness. In *The Clinical Science of Electroconvulsive Therapy* (ed. C. E. Coffey), pp. 183–212. Washington, DC: American Psychiatric Press.

Krishnamoorthy, E. S. & Trimble, M. R. (1999) Forced normalization: clinical and therapeutic relevance. *Epilepsia*, **40** (suppl. 10), S57–S64.

Krystal, A. D. & Coffey, C. E. (1997) Neuropsychiatric considerations in the use of electroconvulsive therapy. *Journal of Neuropsychiatry and Clinical Neurosciences*, **9**, 283–292.

Maltbie, A. A., Wingfield, M. S., Volow, M. R., et al (1980) Electroconvulsive therapy in the presence of brain tumor – case reports and an evaluation of risk. *Journal of Nervous and Mental Disease*, **168**, 400–405.

Meduna, L. (1935) Verushe uber die biologische Beeinflussung des Ablaufes der Schizophrenic. I. Campher- und Cardiazol-Krampfe. *Zeitschrift ges Neurol. Psychiatr*, **152**, 235–262.

Moellentine, C., Rummans, T., Ahlskog, J. E., et al (1998) Effectiveness of ECT in patients with parkinsonism. *Journal of Neuropsychiatry and Clinical Neurosciences*, **10**, 187–193.

Murray, G., Shea, V. & Conn, D. (1986) Electroconvulsive therapy for post-stroke depression. *Journal of Clinical Psychiatry*, **47**, 258–260.

Price, T. R. P. & McAllister, T. W. (1989) Safety and efficacy of ECT in depressed patients with dementia: a review of clinical experience. *Convulsive Therapy*, **5**, 61–74.

Pridmore, S. & Pollard, C. (1996) Electroconvulsive therapy in Parkinson's disease: 30 month follow up. *Journal of Neurology, Neurosurgery and Psychiatry*, **61**, 693.

Rasmussen, K. & Abrams, R. (1991) Treatment of Parkinson's disease with ECT. *Psychiatric Clinics of North America*, **14**, 925–933.

Sackeim, H., Decina, P., Provohnik, I., et al (1983) Anticonvulsant and antidepressant properties of electroconvulsive therapy: a proposed mechanism of action. *Biological Psychiatry*, **18**, 1301–1309.

Sackeim, H., Decina, P., Provohnik, I., et al (1987a) Seizure threshold in electroconvulsive therapy: effects of age, sex, electrode placement, and number of treatments. *Archives of General Psychiatry*, **44**, 355–360.

Sackeim, H., Decina, P., Portnoy, S., et al (1987b) Studies of dosage, seizure threshold, and seizure duration in ECT. *Biological Psychiatry*, **22**, 249–268.

Starkstein, S. E. & Migliorelli, R. (1993) ECT in a patient with a frontal craniotomy and residual meningioma. *Journal of Neuropsychiatry and Clinical Neurosciences*, **5**, 428–430.

Trimble, M. R. (1996) *Biological Psychiatry* (2nd edn). Chichester: Wiley.

Weiner, R. D. & Coffey, C. E. (1993) Electroconvulsive therapy in the medical and neurologic patient. In *Psychiatric Care of the Medical Patient* (ed. A. Stoudemire & B. S. Fogel), pp. 207–224. New York: Oxford University Press.

Zervas, L. & Fink, M. (1991) ECT for refractory Parkinson's disease. *Convulsive Therapy*, **7**, 222–223.

CHAPTER 6

The use of ECT in people with learning disability

Walter J. Muir

'Learning disability' is a descriptive term, not a condition in itself, and although the number of identifiable disorders that alter neurodevelopment and create an associated learning disability is steadily increasing, we are only beginning to understand the many ways in which the altered neural substrate modifies the course and presentation of coexisting psychiatric disorders. Save in the case of relatively common conditions, such as Down's syndrome or fragile X syndrome, studies in learning disability usually involve patients with ill-defined, hetero-geneous aetiologies grouped on the basis of their degree of intellectual impairment rather than proximate causes. It is clear, however, that adults with a learning disability are susceptible to the whole range of psychiatric disorders seen in the general population.

Relative to the use of psychotropic medication, the use of ECT for patients who have both a learning disability and a psychiatric disorder remains uncommon. Research in this area is sparse, as reflected in the fact that much of the relevant literature can be described within this short chapter. Most studies are single case reports or small series and, to my knowledge, there have been no properly randomised clinical trials of the use of ECT in this group, whether blind, open, crossover or parallel controlled. This overview is therefore largely descriptive.

In spite of the scarcity of reports, ECT has a long history of use in patients with learning disability. Bender (1970, 1973) conducted a long-term outcome study on 100 children with 'childhood schizo-phrenia' who were patients of the Bellevue Hospital in New York during the period 1935–52. Diagnostically we would now see this group as suffering from a mixture of unrelated disorders, including autism. A large proportion of the 63 most chronically institutionalised children had a learning disability, ranging from mild to very severe. Fifty-nine of the total received ECT and a further 28 metrazole-induced convulsive therapy. The reports of subsequent clinical improvement are unfor-tunately difficult to interpret in the light of more recent views on the aetiology of these conditions.

Payne (1968) described the use of ECT in a man with a moderate learning disability (and another patient who may well not have had a learning disability) and Reid (1972), in his series of 21 patients with manic–depressive psychosis, felt that both antidepressants and ECT were effective in those with mild learning disability, but that the illness was self-limiting in those with more severe learning disability.

More recently Cutajar & Wilson (1999) received 24 replies to a questionnaire sent to 26 consultant psychiatrists working with people with a learning disability in the Trent region of the UK (population 4.7 million) during the years 1990–95. A (small) majority of respondents felt that ECT was underused in this group and the main reason for this centred on consent issues and diagnostic difficulties. Sayal & Bernard (1998) similarly reported that trainee psychiatrists were less likely to suggest ECT for depressive illness for vignettes of cases of mild learning disability, even though they diagnosed psychotic depression more frequently in this group.

Affective disorder in patients with learning disability and the use of ECT

Prevalence figures for major depressive disorder in people with a learning disability vary from 1% to 5%; diagnostic difficulties contribute to this uncertainty but it is likely that the lower figures are an underestimate. The presentation of illness can be much modified by the degree of intellectual impairment, and with affective disorders as much reliance is placed on observable biological features – such as cyclical mood swings or behavioural change, motor retardation, reduction in the use of speech (mutism in some cases), disturbance of sleep pattern, weight change, apparent loss of day-to-day living skills or decrease in self-care (including continence) and obvious low affect and crying – as on subjective symptoms such as self-expressed low mood and guilt. It is known that people with a learning disability are much less likely to complain directly of psychological symptoms, although they often somatise their complaints, and the observations of change by carers is crucial to diagnosis. People with a severe learning disability may completely lack the verbal skills needed to express their affect and their distress may be conveyed in other ways, such as screaming, aggressive outbursts or self-injury. In this group, suicide and suicidal ideation are rare, but not unknown. This probably does not indicate a lack of severe depression but instead the lack of the complex cognition and communication skills needed to express such feelings. Ballinger's (1997) overview of the presentation of affective disorders in patients with a learning disability covers all these areas.

In Cutajar & Wilson's series, eight patients (four with mild and four with moderate learning disability) had received ECT (laterality not stated) during the period – a low rate compared with other areas of psychiatry. A brief synopsis is given for only four of these patients, but mention is made that the best responses were when biological features of depression and psychotic features predominated (six of the eight). Thuppal & Fink (1999) reported that psychotic features were also present in a male patient with mild learning disability and major depressive disorder who received several sessions of bilateral ECT in combination with a neuroleptic (trifluoperazine) and in addition maintenance ECT; the patient's last session of ECT was limited by physical complications but seemed to have a mood-elevating effect. In another report (Goldstein & Jensvold, 1989) post-surgical deterioration in an elderly man with mild learning disability and depression seemed to be reversed by unilateral ECT. Depressive illness in another older patient (a 67-year-old woman with mild learning disability) with bipolar affective disorder was said to have had a good response to nine sessions of ECT and to a further 12 sessions after a relapse two months later (Van Waarde et al, 2001).

Persistent screaming is a distressing symptom that may be unrelated in some cases to depression. However, where other evidence for a depressive disorder exists, such as in the case of an elderly woman with mild learning disability, (unilateral and bilateral) ECT has been used effectively (Snowdon et al, 1994). Jancar & Gunaratne (1994) described two patients with episodes of major depressive disorder with psychotic features who also had chronic dysthymia. In a man with moderate learning disability, the major depressive episodes responded to ECT (laterality not stated) but not his persistent nihilistic and hypochondriacal delusions. In a woman with mild learning disability, paranoid and hypochondriacal delusions were said to respond to ECT but not her depressed mood. Cutajar et al (1998) also described a woman with a mild learning disability who developed an ECT-responsive post-partum depressive disorder.

None of the patients in these reports had a severe learning disability and in the past it has been argued that severe learning disability and depression are mutually exclusive. Current opinion would not favour this view, and the main issue in treatment of this group is again of consent. Bates & Smeltzer (1982) in Ohio used bilateral ECT in a patient with severe learning disability, pervasive developmental disorder and treatment-refractory self-injury to such an incessant degree that it endangered life. Judicial authorisation (in essence a law change) was required for a course of six sessions of ECT, which was followed by effective control with lithium. That self-injury in this case might have been a manifestation of an underlying depressive illness is hinted at by the family history of bipolar disorder. Repeated treatment-refractory self-injurious behaviour occurs more frequently in patients with severe learning disability and is probably one of the most distressing conditions that face the psychiatrist. Fink (1999) reported another success in treating severe repetitive self-injurious behaviour in a child of 14 years with moderate learning disability. Twice-weekly maintenance therapy was continued to a total of 16 treatments. Merrill (1990) reported the case of a treatment-refractory patient who had severe learning disability with cycles of severe agitated behaviour, including self-injury requiring physical restraint. Judicial approval allowed treatment with a course of six sessions of ECT (laterality not stated), which resulted in marked improvement. Judicial approval was also required for the use of unilateral ECT in a patient with bipolar disorder, cerebral palsy and a mild learning disability (Guze *et al*, 1987) who subsequently had a manic episode questionably related to the therapy (six weeks after ECT).

Delusions may be a prominent feature in patients with depression and mild to moderate learning disability who have the required communication skills and, as in the general population, psychotic features may predict a better response to ECT. Fixed nihilistic delusions observed in a man with moderate to severe learning disability and depressed mood responded to ECT (laterality not stated) (Kearns, 1987). In the case of a man with moderate learning disability and strikingly similar nihilistic delusions, out-patient bilateral ECT was successful (Kavournis *et al*, 1992).

ECT in syndromic conditions associated with learning disability

There is some evidence that Down's syndrome is associated with an increased risk of depression, especially for women and those in their third decade. Adults with Down's syndrome are also at increased risk of medical and psychological complications whose symptoms can mimic depression – for example, hypothyroidism is very common and some-times undetected, and bereavement reactions can be particularly intense (partly because the parents are often older and tend to continue to care for their adult children with learning disability). Although dementia is significantly more frequent in older adults with Down's syndrome, and depression is a key differential diagnosis, it is comparatively rare in those under the age of 40 years.

Of five patients aged 17–38 years with Down's syndrome referred to Warren *et al* (1989) for evaluation of apparent dementia, all had major depressive disorder, psychotic features were described in four, and ECT (laterality not stated) was used successfully in three who were either treatment refractory or showed unacceptable side-effects from medica-tion. Lazarus *et al* (1990) described two women with Down's syndrome who had mild learning disability as well as treatment-refractory/ recurrent major depressive disorder. Both responded to bilateral ECT; one went on to have maintenance ECT and the other had received this in the past. It should be mentioned here that a few people with Down's syndrome have instability of the atlanto-axial neck joint. Although this rarely limits an active life, there have been undetected cases where manipulation or restraint has led to severe injury or death, and the anaesthetist who is performing ECT should be aware of these risks, especially relating to intubation and muscle relaxation.

Very little had been published about the use of ECT in other syndromes that have learning disability as a component. Gotholf *et al* (1999) noted that the psychotic symptoms of one of their patients who had a mild learning disability, chronic schizophrenia and the velocardio-facial syndrome (microdeletion within the long arm of chromosome 22) had not responded to repeated courses of ECT. The co-occurrence of learning disability in a man who developed the extremely rare adult-onset form of Tay–Sach's disease (GM_2 gangliosidosis) may be coincidental (Renshaw *et al*, 1992). His severe depression responded to unilateral ECT and fluoxetine.

ECT for other psychiatric disorders in people with learning disability

In addition to depression, ECT has been used to control manic episodes. ECT (laterality not stated) was used to control treatment-resistant mania in a patient with mild learning disability (Everman & Stoudemire, 1994), although it had been ineffective in a similar case with neuroleptic malignant syndrome described previously by the same group (Slack & Stoudemire, 1989). ECT was also used after the appearance of neuroleptic malignant syndrome by Aziz *et al* (2001) – a man with bipolar affective disorder and moderate learning disability successfully re-sponded to a series of six bilateral ECT sessions over the course of 2 weeks. In Thuppal & Fink's series (1999) one man with moderate learning disability had behavioural symptoms of decreased sleep, agitation and periods of excitability with assaults on staff. These were unresponsive to a variety of neuroleptics, including clozapine, and mood stabilisers, including carbamazepine and valproate. A course of 13 sessions of bilateral ECT produced a marked improvement. Four sessions of out-patient continuation ECT were given after discharge. Clozapine was continued throughout.

Jyoti Rao *et al* (1993) reported the case of an 18-year-old man with moderate learning disability where treatment for a non-organic psy-chosis (diagnosis not further specified) with a course of ECT incurred the rare complication of non-convulsive status epilepticus during the ninth treatment. They argued for intratreatment electroencephalo-graphic monitoring, which would seem a sensible general precaution.

Symptoms of schizophrenia in people with learning disability have also been treated with ECT (see next section). It has also been used to treat a variety of less well-defined psychiatric syndromes, including catatonic states. Zaw *et al* (1999) treated a 14-year-old boy with moderate learning disability, autism and a catatonic stupor that required him to have nasogastric nutrition and fluid replacement. There were affective components to his illness but standard antidepressant treatment had not helped and zolpidem produced only a temporary improvement in the catatonia. Bilateral ECT produced a significant response after the third treatment, and progressive improvement to the end of the course of 13 sessions. Successful maintenance on a neuroleptic–lithium combination and previous episodes of catatonic excitement are suggestive of an underlying bipolar disorder in this case. A clearer link is shown by Finks' (1999) description of a patient with a moderate learning disability where catatonia coexisted with bipolar (mixed affective) disorder. ECT followed by maintenance ECT produced symptom allevi-ation without the need for continuation of psychotropic drugs. Thuppal & Fink (1999) described an adult with mild learning disability and a schizophrenic illness with catatonia to whom intravenous fluids had to be given. The catatonia responded to six sessions of bilateral ECT, but he required a further 45 sessions as maintenance therapy over 7 months. Another patient with moderate learning disability and a bipolar disorder poorly controlled by medication was treated with bilateral ECT during a depressed phase with marked lorazepam-responsive catatonic features. Again, maintenance therapy was used (31 sessions over 9 months). Aziz *et al* (2001) reported the case of a woman aged 39 years with moderate learning disability who had a schizoaffective disorder with marked catatonic features. A marked improvement was seen in the catatonic symptoms after five sessions of bilateral ECT in an eventual course of 11 treatments. One of Cutajar & Wilson's (1999) patients had autism and received ECT for catatonia without effect.

The use of ECT as a maintenance therapy

Maintenance bilateral ECT (given on average every third week for over a year) was said to be useful in the treatment of a relapsing depression with psychotic features in a man with mild learning disability (Puri *et al*, 1992). In another case, a woman with a mild learning disability and recurrent psychotic depression improved with a course of sessions of ECT followed by another seven after a relapse (Ruedrich & Alamir, 1999); monthly maintenance ECT was then instigated over a 2-year period. Gabriel (1998) used maintenance ECT (laterality not stated) in a woman aged 65 years who had chronic, treatment-refractory schizophrenia and was also said to have a moderate learning disability. Twice-weekly ECT (30 treatments) was followed by maintenance on a 7–10-day interval schedule. This is one of the few reports that feature the use of structured ratings to detail response to ECT. The patient's score on the Brief Psychological Rating Scale decreased and the Global Assessment of Function score increased significantly from baseline. It is not stated whether this was maintained.

Combined maintenance bilateral ECT and flupenthixol therapy was used in three patients with moderate to severe learning disability to control psychotic symptoms (Chanpattana, 1999). Two were said to conform to DSM–IV criteria for schizophrenia and the third was given a diagnosis of paranoid schizophrenia. Owing to the pleiomorphic nature of psychosis in people with more severe learning disabilities, there must be some caution regarding the diagnosis, but the psychotic symptoms were largely persecutory. Bebchuk et al (1996) also describe problems in differential diagnosis (between major depressive disorder, bipolar disorder and dementia) in a man with profound learning disability. It is of note that episodic self-injury was a feature of his condition. The early rapid response to ECT (unilateral) and monthly maintenance ECT was followed by a relapse and the instigation of a course of bilateral ECT and twice-weekly maintenance out-patient therapy of unspecified duration with reported success.

Observations on reported usage

Only Cutajar & Wilson's (1999) study looked at features of actual practice. All others are case reports. It is impossible to say whether these reflect general practice in the field, but selective and biased reporting is probably inevitable. With such caveats in mind, some tentative points may be made:

- The use of ECT seems to be much less frequent in adults with a learning disability than among other sections of the population.
- The presence of learning disability of any degree, however, has not been a contraindication to the use of ECT.
- As in the case in the general population, its use has not been restricted to the treatment of depressive disorders.
- Most descriptions are of patients whose psychiatric disorder has failed to respond to medication or of patients who exhibit life-threatening behaviours.
- Many reports note its efficacy where psychotic features are present, which would accord with findings in the general population.
- Maintenance ECT is reported in a surprisingly large proportion of cases.

- Where the laterality is stated, bilateral ECT is by far the most frequently used.
- In the majority of reports there are no indications of how improvement after ECT was measured, and this lack of outcome data is especially relevant when the frequency of maintenance use is considered.

Cognitive adverse effects

Concerns about the side-effects of ECT are highly relevant to people with learning disability, who have much less functional reserve to cope with any additional cognitive impairment. The current views on cognitive side-effects have been summarised by Sackeim (2000). The degree of profound short- and long-term retrograde amnesia is related to the degree of preictal global cognitive impairment (for example as rated on the modified Mini-Mental State Examination) in those without a learning disability. None of the reports of the use of ECT for people with a learning disability prospectively featured objective measures of functioning that included tests of memory, either before treatment or over the course of treatment and recovery. There are psychological instruments validated in this population that could be used. Objective clinical measures of recovery and outcome, essential for the valid comparison of different studies, are also rarely used. These points are further highlighted by the number of reports describing maintenance therapy without measures of cognitive or clinical outcome. Justification for the predominant use of bilateral ECT is usually not stated. Evidence does suggest that high-dose unilateral ECT may be as effective as bilateral placement and produces fewer cognitive side-effects. One possible confounder here is the very high prevalence of epilepsy in adults with learning disability. This is certainly not a contraindication to ECT, but the often complex anticonvulsant therapeutic regimens may alter the ECT seizure threshold.

Consent

The legal issues of consent are complex and differ in different areas of the UK (see Chapter 20). It can be simply mentioned that adults with moderate to severe degrees of learning disability nearly always lack the ability to give full informed consent, but mild learning disability in itself (rather than the effects of a coexisting psychiatric illness) is not necessarily a barrier to informed consent, provided sufficient thought has gone into how the information is given to the person, and how the person's understanding of that information is ascertained.

Note added in proof

Since this chapter was written some further (retrospective) reports have been published on the use of ECT in people with learning disability. The recommendations given are not changed, only strengthened by these. Friedlander & Solomons (2002) retrospectively reviewed the clinical details of ten patients who received ECT who had learning disability of varied severity comorbid with a number of different severe affective illnesses. Retrospective scores on the Clinical Global Impressions (CGI) scale were used to judge outcome and all were treated with bilateral ECT. It was noted that good responders (7 out of 10) tended to have a very rapid response, within the first few treatments. Two patients whose schizoaffective disorder was accompanied by catatonia responded less well. Interestingly three patients with bipolar disorder, either manic or mixed type, showed a good response. Little *et al* (2002) reported three further cases with psychotic depression. All were initially given bilateral ECT with effect, and one was subsequently given unilateral ECT also with clinical improvement. In reviewing the literature they stressed the frequent delay in using ECT that appeared to arise from various and sometimes misguided ethical concerns. As a consequence ECT often emerges as a treatment of last resort. Reinblatt *et al* (2004) retrospectively analysed a larger case series of 20 individuals with learning disability of varying severity, who received bitemporal or bifrontal ECT. Aberrant behaviour checklist (ABC) scores were available and CGI scores created, and all had failed previous trials of behaviour therapy and pharmacotherapy. The diagnostic groupings were broad (12 with 'mood disorders' - bipolar disorders and major depression; 6 with 'psychotic disorders' – schizoaffective disorder and schizophrenia; 2 with intermittent explosive disorder), but overall response was good for mood and psychotic disorders, with decreases in ABC subscores for hyperactivity and irritability being especially notable. In contrast the two subjects with intermittent explosive disorder showed no clinical improvement and, in fact, a worsening on the ABC hyperactivity subscale.

Recommendations

- There have been no randomised controlled trials specifically in people with learning disability.
- It would be good practice to use ECT only in carefully selected cases, usually where the psychiatric illness has proved refractory to medical treatment or where there are intolerable adverse effects of medication, or where the clinical condition of the sufferer has severely deteriorated.

- There are no absolute contraindications to the use of ECT in patients with a learning disability.

References

Aziz, M., Maixner, D. F., DeQuardo, J., *et al* (2001) ECT and mental retardation: a review and case reports. *Journal of ECT*, **17**, 149–152.

Ballinger, C. B. (1997) Affective disorders. In *Psychiatry in Learning Disability* (ed. S. G. Read), pp 216–236. London: Saunders.

Bates, W. J. & Smeltzer, M. A. (1982) Electroconvulsive treatment of psychotic self-injurious behavior in a patient with severe mental retardation. *American Journal of Psychiatry*, **139**, 1355–1356.

Bebchuk, J. M., Barnhill, J. & Dawkins, K. (1996) ECT and mental retardation. *American Journal of Psychiatry*, **153**, 1231.

Bender, L. (1970) The life course of schizophrenic children. *Biological Psychiatry*, **2**, 165–172.

Bender, L. (1973) The life course of children with schizophrenia. *American Journal of Psychiatry*, **130**, 783–786.

Chanpattana, W. (1999) Maintenance ECT in mentally retarded treatment-resistant schizophrenic patients. *Journal of ECT*, **15**, 150–153.

Cutajar, P. & Wilson, D. (1999) The use of ECT in intellectual disability. *Journal of Intellectual Disability Research*, **43**, 421–427.

Cutajar, P., Wilson, D. N. & Mukherjee, T. (1998) ECT used in depression following childbirth, in a woman with learning disabilities. *British Journal of Learning Disabilities*, **26**, 115–117.

Everman, D. B. & Stoudemire, A. (1994) Bipolar disorder associated with Klinefelter's syndrome and other chromosomal abnormalities. *Psychosomatics*, **35**, 35–40.

Fink, M. (1999) *Electroshock, Restoring the Mind*. Oxford: Oxford University Press.

Friedlander, R. I. & Solomons, K. (2002) ECT: use in individuals with mental retardation. *Journal of ECT*, **18**, 38–42.

Gabriel, A. (1998) ECT and maintenance in a patient with psychosis and mental disability. *Canadian Journal of Psychiatry*, **43**, 305–306.

Goldstein, M. Z. & Jensvold, M. F. (1989) ECT treatment of an elderly mentally retarded man. *Psychosomatics*, **30**, 104–106.

Gothelf, D., Frisch, A., Munitz, H., *et al* (1999) Clinical characteristics of schizophrenia associated with velo-cardio-facial syndrome. *Schizophrenia Research*, **35**, 105–112.

Guze, B. H., Weinman, B. & Diamond, R. P. (1987) Use of ECT to treat bipolar depression in a mental retardate with cerebral palsy. *Convulsive Therapy*, **3**, 60–64.

Jancar, J. & Gunaratne, I. J. (1994) Dysthymia and mental handicap. *British Journal of Psychiatry*, **164**, 691–693.

Jyoti Rao, K. M. J., Gandahar, B. N. & Janakirmaiah, N. (1993) Nonconvulsive status epilepticus after the ninth electroconvulsive therapy. *Convulsive Therapy*, **9**, 128–129.

Kavournis, S., Holt, G. & Hodgkiss, A. (1992) Out-patient ECT for depression in a man with moderate learning disability (letter). *British Journal of Psychiatry*, **161**, 426–427.

Kearns, A. (1987) Cotard's syndrome in a mentally handicapped man. *British Journal of Psychiatry*, **150**, 112–114.

Lazarus, A., Jaffe, R. L. & Dubin, W. R. (1990) Electroconvulsive therapy and major depression in Down's syndrome. *Journal of Clinical Psychiatry*, **51**, 422–425.

Little, J. D., McFarlane, J. & Ducharme, H. M. (2002) ECT use delayed in the presence of comorbid mental retardation: a review of clinical and ethical issues. *Journal of ECT*, **18**, 218–222.

Merrill, R. D. (1990) ECT for a patient with profound mental retardation. *American Journal of Psychiatry*, **147**, 256–257.

Payne, R. (1968) The psychotic subnormal. *Journal of Mental Subnormality*, **139**, 1355–1356.

Puri, B. K., Langa, A., Coleman, R. M., *et al* (1992) The clinical efficacy of maintenance electroconvulsive therapy in a patient with mild mental handicap. *British Journal of Psychiatry*, **161**, 707–709.

Reid, A. H. (1972) Psychoses in adult mental defectives, I: manic depressive psychosis. *British Journal of Psychiatry*, **120**, 205–212.

Reinblatt, S. P., Rifkin, A. & Freeman, J. (2004) The efficacy of ECT in adults with mental retardation experiencing psychiatric disorders. *Journal of ECT*, **20**, 208–212.

Renshaw, P. R., Stern, T. A., Welch, C., *et al* (1992) Electroconvulsive therapy treatment of depression in a patient with adult GM_2 gangliosidosis. *Annals of Neurology*, **31**, 342–344.

Ruedrich, S. L. & Alamir, S. (1999) Electroconvulsive therapy for persons with developmental disabilities: review, case report and recommendations. *Mental Health Aspects of Developmental Disability*, **2**, 83–91.

Sackeim, H. A. (2000) Memory and ECT: from polarization to reconciliation. *Journal of ECT*, **16**, 87–96.

Sayal, K. & Bernard S. (1998) Trainees' assessment and management of mental illness in adults with mild learning disability. *Psychiatric Bulletin*, **22**, 571–572.

Slack, T. & Stoudemire, A. (1989) Reinstitution of neuroleptic treatment with molindone in a patient with a history of neuroleptic malignant syndrome. *General Hospital Psychiatry*, **11**, 365–367.

Snowdon, J., Meehan, T. & Halpin, R. (1994) Continuous screaming controlled by electroconvulsive therapy: a case study. *International Journal of Geriatric Psychiatry*, **9**, 929–932.

Thuppal, M. & Fink, M. (1999) Electroconvulsive therapy and mental retardation. *Journal of ECT*, **15**, 140–149.

Van Waarde, J. A., Stolker, J. J. & van der Mast, R. C. (2001) ECT in mental retardation: a review. *Journal of ECT*, **17**, 236–243.

Warren, A. C., Holroyd, S. & Folstein, M. F. (1989) Major depression in Down's syndrome. *British Journal of Psychiatry*, **155**, 202–205.

Zaw, F. K. M., Bates, G. D. L., Murali, V., *et al* (1999) Catatonia, autism and ECT. *Developmental Medicine and Child Neurology*, **41**, 843–845.

CHAPTER 7

Safe ECT practice in people with a physical illness

Susan M. Benbow

Possible medical contraindications to ECT

People with a wide range of physical illnesses are successfully treated with ECT (Fink, 1999; American Psychiatric Association, 2001). Abrams (1997) pointed out that the death rate associated with ECT is lower than the spontaneous death rate in the general US population. Some medical problems may cause particular concern, however, especially cardiovascular and neurological problems.

During the passage of the electrical stimulus, both blood pressure and heart rate fall and then rise rapidly. There is a sudden, short-lived rise in intracranial pressure and cerebral blood flow, and cerebrovascular permeability increases. Vagal stimulation leads to a sinus bradycardia, sometimes with periods of asystole, or electrical silence. This is rapidly replaced by a sympathetically mediated tachycardia, which, by decreasing the oxygen supply to the myocardium and increasing its oxygen consumption, increases cardiac work and can result in ischaemia. Subconvulsive stimuli are known to produce longer periods of brady-cardia; this may be a concern when people with established heart disease are being treated using a dose-titration protocol to determine seizure threshold (Abrams, 1991; Dolinski & Zvara, 1997). Another risk factor for longer periods of asystole during ECT is the use of beta-blockers (McCall, 1996). Vagolytic drugs, such as glycopyrrolate and atropine, are sometimes used to attenuate the bradycardia (Applegate, 1997).

Thus, it is not surprising that there is evidence that people with cardiovascular disease have been shown to be at increased risk of cardiac complications during ECT. Burke et al (1987) reported more complications in people on a greater total number of medications and in those on a greater number of cardiovascular medications. Complications during ECT may also increase as the age of the person being treated increases, although, in a naturalistic study, Brodaty et al (2000) found that the number and severity of adverse events were not associated with age. Most cardiovascular complications are transient and do not prevent successful completion of the course of treatment, and so Zielinski *et al* (1998) concluded that ECT can still be used relatively safely for people with severe cardiac disease. The American Psychiatric Association (2001) also states that, in general, people with cardiovascular disease can be safely treated with ECT. Abrams (2002) has reviewed the use of ECT in people with previous cardiac surgery, myocardial infarction, cardiac pacemakers, aortic aneurysms and intracardiac thrombi, and who were taking drug treatments to reduce blood pressure, prevent arrhythmias or reduce heart rate. He noted that the 'detection and management of significant cardiovascular disease before administering ECT … is … the most important factor in reducing … cardiovascular morbidity and mortality'.

Coexisting medical or surgical conditions

Since many medical illnesses could increase the risk associated with ECT, it is important that all people for whom ECT is being considered are fully evaluated before treatment. Any physical illness will need to be investigated and treated or at least stabilised as far as possible before ECT is begun. The important principles here are as follows:

- When a person who is being considered for treatment with ECT is thought to present high risk, an appropriate medical opinion should be sought to clarify the degree of risk and ways of minimising that risk.
- Any underlying disorder will be fully assessed and treated before ECT.
- An anaesthetic opinion may also be sought at this stage and, in liaison with the anaesthetist, treatment technique may be modified to minimise the risks involved.
- During the consent process, patient and family should be informed of the increased risk and any recommendations for minimising it. Risk may need to be reassessed following cardiological or anaesthetic opinion or investigation.
- High-risk patients will not normally be treated at remote sites, or as day patients or out-patients.

Cardiovascular disease

Electroconvulsive therapy is classed as a low-risk procedure (Applegate, 1997) but, although it is quite unlike other procedures for which a general anaesthetic is administered, the conditions that may present higher cardiac risks during treatment are likely to be similar to those that elevate the risks associated with surgical interventions (Dolinski & Zvara, 1997), and include the following:

- recent myocardial infarct (for advice regarding management, see Applegate, 1997)
- severe valvular heart disease (for a review, see Rayburn, 1997; for case reports, see Rasmussen, 1997)
- clinically significant cardiac dysrhythmias (for advice regarding management, see Applegate, 1997)
- unstable angina (for advice regarding management, see Applegate, 1997)
- uncompensated congestive cardiac failure (for a review, see Rayburn, 1997)
- some aneurysms (for a case report of left ventricular aneurysm, see Gardner *et al*, 1997).

Neurological conditions

Electroconvulsive therapy has been used safely for people with small, slow-growing cerebral tumours without raised intracranial pressure, but people who have space-occupying lesions of the brain are at high risk of neurological deterioration if treated with ECT (Krystal & Coffey, 1997). The aggravation of already raised intracranial pressure is thought to account for the risk (Abrams, 2002). Nevertheless, people with a wide range of neurological conditions have been treated successfully with ECT. This includes the following groups :

- people with cerebrovascular diseases (for a review of cerebral aneurysm and case reports, see Bader *et al*, 1995; for a review of cerebrovascular disease and ECT and case reports of reversible ischaemic neurological deficit after ECT, see Miller & Isenberg, 1998)
- people with epilepsy (for a review, see Hsiao *et al*, 1987)
- people with cerebral lupus (for a review, see Hsiao *et al*, 1987)
- people with dementia, including advanced dementia (for a case report, see Weintraub & Lippmann, 2001; and for a report of a retrospective series, see Rao & Lyketsos, 2000)
- people with learning disability (for case reports, see Thuppal & Fink, 1999; for a review and case reports, see Aziz *et al*, 2001) (see also Chapter 6)
- those who have had a stroke (for a review, see Gustafson *et al*, 1995)
- those who have undergone craniotomy (for a review and a case report, see Gursky *et al*, 2000).

Other medical conditions

The anaesthetist should be informed of all relevant medical and surgical conditions before treatment and of any conditions developing or diagnosed during treatment. The anaesthetist will advise on any special precautions; for example, since oesophageal reflux is associated with an increased risk of aspiration during ECT, measures to decrease or neutralise gastric acidity may be necessary, as may modifications to anaesthetic technique (Bowley & Walker, 2005). The patient's management of diabetes may need to be modified (Weiner & Sibert, 1996). People with bone or joint disease may need an increased dose of muscle relaxant, although fracture during ECT has been virtually eliminated with the use of muscle-relaxant drugs (American Psychiatric Association, 2001). Ophthalmological advice should be sought in people with advanced glaucoma (Abrams, 2002) in view of the transient rise in intra-occular pressure during ECT. The American Psychiatric Association (2001) gave detailed advice regarding cardiovascular, neurological and other disorders, but the principles of good practice are common to all.

Minimising risk

When a person is thought to be at greater risk because of a coexisting medical or surgical condition, consideration should always be given to ways of minimising risk by modifying medical management or ECT technique. High-risk patients should not be treated at remote sites or as out-patients. Modifications to medical treatment or ECT technique will require liaison between anaesthetist, psychiatrist and any other specialist involved. Some people at high risk may best be treated in a cardiac care unit, with ECG monitoring before, during and after the treatment and with specialist staff to hand who are trained in cardio-pulmonary resuscitation and the emergency treatment of arrhythmias.

Balance of risks and benefits

The balance of risks and benefits to physical and mental health must be considered for each individual. The risk–benefit analysis will include the following considerations:

- the severity of the psychiatric illness and the risks it poses to the individual
- the likelihood of the psychiatric illness responding to ECT
- the medical risks of ECT and the extent to which they can be minimised or controlled
- options for alternative treatments, the likely response to and adverse effects of those treatments, and the likely outcome if the person opts for no treatment.

The patient and family will normally be fully involved in discussions relating to the risk–benefit analysis. Where a person is detained under the Mental Health Act and is unable to give consent, it is good practice to involve the relatives fully during assessment and before invoking the 'second opinion' procedure.

Involving families

As far as is practicable, patients and their families should be involved in discussions about the treatment, its risks, its possible benefits and alternatives. Where the risk of ECT remains high, the patient and, where appropriate, the family should be informed and then involved in the careful balancing of risks and benefits.

Recommendations

- The balance of risks and benefits to physical and mental health must be considered for each individual.
- As far as possible, patients and, where appropriate, their families should be involved in discussions about the treatment, its risks, its possible benefits and any alternative treatments.
- All coexisting medical or surgical conditions should be assessed and, where possible, treated or stabilised before ECT is administered.
- When a patient is thought to be at greater risk during ECT, consideration should always be given to ways of minimising risk by modifying medical management or ECT technique (or both).
- On the occasions when ECT is prescribed to save life, there may be no absolute contraindications to it.

References

Abrams, R. (1991) Electroconvulsive therapy in the medically compromised patient. *Psychiatric Clinics of North America*, **14**, 871–885.

Abrams, R. (1997) The mortality rate with ECT. *Convulsive Therapy*, **13**, 125–127.

Abrams, R. (2002) Electroconvulsive therapy in the high-risk patient. In *Electroconvulsive Therapy* (4th edn), pp. 72–100. New York: Oxford University Press.

American Psychiatric Association (2001) *The Practice of Electroconvulsive Therapy: Recommendations for Treatment, Training and Privileging* (2nd edn). Washington, DC: APA.

Applegate, R. J. (1997) Diagnosis and management of ischaemic heart disease in the patient scheduled to undergo electroconvulsive therapy. *Convulsive Therapy*, **13**, 128–144.

Aziz, M., Maixner, D. F., Dequardo, J., *et al* (2001) ECT and mental retardation: a review and case reports. *Journal of ECT*, **17**, 149–152.

Bader, G. M., Silk, K. R., Dequardo, J. R., *et al* (1995) Electroconvulsive therapy and intracranial aneurysm. *Convulsive Therapy*, **11**, 139–143.

Bowley, C. J. & Walker, H. A. C. (2005) Anaesthesia for ECT. In *The ECT Handbook*, 2nd edn. (ed. A. I. F. Scott), pp. 124–135. Council Report CR128. London: Royal College of Psychiatrists.

Brodaty, H., Hickie, I., Mason, C., *et al* (2000) A prospective follow-up study of ECT outcome in older depressed patients. *Journal of Affective Disorders*, **60**, 101–111.

Burke, W. J., Rubin, E. H., Zorumski, C. F., *et al* (1987) The safety of ECT in geriatric psychiatry. *Journal of the American Geriatrics Society*, **35**, 516–521.

Dolinski, S. Y. & Zvara, D. A. (1997) Anesthetic considerations of cardiovascular risk during electroconvulsive therapy. *Convulsive Therapy*, **13**, 157–164.

Fink, M. (1999) *Electroshock: Restoring the Mind*. Oxford: Oxford University Press.

Gardner, M. W., Kellner, C. H., Hood, D. E., *et al* (1997) Safe administration of ECT in a patient with a cardiac aneurysm and multiple cardiac risk factors. *Convulsive Therapy*, **13**, 200–203.

Gursky, J. T., Rummans, T. A. & Black, J. L. (2000) ECT administration in a patient after craniotomy and gamma knife surgery: a case report and review. *Journal of ECT*, **16**, 295–299.

Gustafson, Y., Nilsson, I., Mattsson, M., *et al* (1995) Epidemiology and treatment of post-stroke depression. *Drugs and Aging*, **7**, 298–309.

Hsiao, J. K., Messenheimer, J. A. & Evans, D. L. (1987) ECT and neurological disorders. *Convulsive Therapy*, **3**, 121–136.

Krystal, A. D. & Coffey, C. E. (1997) Neuropsychiatric considerations in the use of electroconvulsive therapy. *Journal of Neuropsychiatry and Clinical Neurosciences*, **9**, 283–292.

McCall, W. V. (1996) Asystole in electroconvulsive therapy: report of four cases. *Journal of Clinical Psychiatry*, **5**, 199–203.

Miller, A. R. & Isenberg, K. E. (1998) Reversible ischemic neurologic deficit after ECT. *Journal of ECT*, **14**, 42–48.

Rao, V. & Lyketsos, C. G. (2000) The benefits and risks of ECT for patients with primary dementia who also suffer from depression. *International Journal of Geriatric Psychiatry*, **15**, 729–735.

Rasmussen, K. G. (1997) Electroconvulsive therapy in patients wih aortic stenosis. *Convulsive Therapy*, **13**, 196–199.

Rayburn, B. K. (1997) Electroconvulsive therapy in patients with heart failure or valvular heart disease. *Convulsive Therapy*, **13**, 145–156.

Thuppal, M. & Fink, M. (1999) Electroconvulsive therapy and mental retardation. *Journal of ECT*, **15**, 140–149.

Weiner, R. D. & Sibert, T. E. (1996) Use of ECT in treatment of depression in patients with diabetes mellitus. *Journal of Clinical Psychiatry*, **57**, 138.

Weintraub, D. & Lippmann, S. B. (2001) ECT for major depression and mania with advanced dementia. *Journal of ECT*, **17**, 65–67.

Zielinski, R. J., Roose, S. P., Devanand, D. P., *et al* (1998) Cardiovascular complications of ECT in depressed patients with cardiac disease. *American Journal of Psychiatry*, **150**, 904–909.

CHAPTER 8

The use of ECT for older adults

Susan M. Benbow

Rates of use

The usage of ECT in general adult psychiatry in the UK has fallen significantly since the publication of the first edition of *The ECT Handbook* in 1995 (see also Chapter 2). Such a fall has not been seen in the practice of old age psychiatry, hence the special consideration in this edition to the use of ECT in the elderly person.

Pippard & Ellam (1981) carried out a national survey of ECT usage in Britain and found that 37% of courses were given to people aged over 60 years of age. A total of 137 940 ECT treatments were administered in England in 1985, but usage fell to a reported total of 105 466 treatments in the period 1 April 1990 to 31 March 1991 (220 treatments per 100 000 population) (Department of Health, 1992). A survey of the use of ECT in England in the first quarter of 1999 (Department of Health, 1999) reported a total of 16 500 treatments administered to 2800 individuals (extrapolating from these figures gives a full-year estimate of around 66 000 treatments in England). People aged over 65 years accounted for 44% of the women treated and 33% of the men. Thus people aged over 65 are major users of English ECT services. Similarly in Wales, Duffett *et al* (1999) surveyed the use of ECT and found that people aged over 65 were 2.25 times more likely to receive ECT than people aged 20–64 years. Findings in the United States are similar (Kramer, 1987; Olfson *et al*, 1998; Reid *et al*, 1998).

The mental health charity Mind has argued that older women are over-represented among the population of people treated with ECT, and has campaigned for a scaling down of its use (Cobb, 1995). However, there are several possible reasons why older people might be more likely to require ECT. They may be more likely to suffer from the sorts of illnesses which respond to ECT. Refusal to eat or drink, severe psychosis and stupor may be more common in older age groups. It may also be that depression in later life is more likely to be resistant to drug therapy (Prudic *et al*, 1990). The greater speed of response to ECT may lead to it being used preferentially in people whose physical health exacerbates the urgency of treatment. There may be differences among older patients in their attitudes towards, or acceptance of, ECT. There is some evidence suggesting that older depressed adults may preferentially respond to ECT rather than antidepressant drugs and the response rates quoted in the literature for older adults are around 70% or more (Fraser & Glass, 1980; Gaspar & Samarasinghe, 1982; Karlinsky & Shulman, 1984; Benbow, 1987; Godber *et al*, 1987; Rubin *et al*, 1991; Casey & Davies, 1996; Tomac *et al*, 1997).

It has sometimes been assumed that the increased use of ECT in older people might relate to their increased sensitivity to the side-effects of older antidepressants. Olfson *et al* (1998) argue that, with the introduction of newer antidepressant drugs, this can no longer be the case.

Indications for use

Old age psychiatrists regard the main indication for ECT in older people as severe depressive illness (Benbow, 1991), but also rate the treatment as often or sometimes useful in schizoaffective disorder and depressive illness with dementia. Similarly among old age psychiatrists, ECT is regarded as the treatment of choice in the following depressive illnesses: those that have failed to respond to antidepressant drugs; those in which previous episodes responded to ECT but not to antidepressant drugs; those with psychotic symptoms; those with severe agitation; and those with high suicidal risk.

Access to ECT among older people

People who might benefit from ECT ought not to be denied treatment solely on the grounds of age. Older people are no less likely to respond to ECT than younger people and are entitled to have access to a treatment that might benefit them. The National Service Farmework for Older People (Department of Health, 2001) states that services will be provided, regardless of age, on the basis of clinical need alone, and that older people should have access to a full range of psychological and physical treatments. This will include access to ECT where appropriate.

Coexisting medical and surgical conditions

When ECT is being considered for an older person, all coexisting medical and surgical conditions should be assessed and, where possible, stabilised or treated before ECT (see Chapter 7). It is important to note that such conditions tend to accumulate with increasing age.

Seizure threshold

There is an increased likelihood of a high seizure threshold in an elderly person, particularly an older man. This may increase the difficulty of eliciting effective seizures (Sackeim *et al*, 1987; Coffey *et al*, 1995; Boylan *et al*, 2000).

The choice of anaesthetic agent will need to take account of this and other age-related factors. The relative merits of various anaesthetic agents in this regard were set out by Freeman (1999) following the withdrawal of methohexitone in the UK. The seizure-shortening effect of propofol and its possible effect on seizure threshold will need to be taken into account in chosing an anaesthetic drug.

ECT clinic treatment protocols should also take the likelihood of a high seizure threshold into account and the choice of anaesthetic agent.

Adverse effects

Zervas *et al* (1993) found that, among people aged 20–65 years, 24–72 hours after ECT memory deficits were more severe in older people and the authors concluded that older people treated with ECT are more vulnerable to the development of cognitive side-effects during treatment and at risk of the cognitive side-effects lasting longer. Although this study excluded people aged over 65 years, it may be reasonable to conclude that they would be at even greater risk of cognitive adverse effects. People who have pre-existing memory problems should likewise be regarded as at higher risk of developing cognitive adverse effects during treatment. In either case, modifications to treatment technique may be indicated, such as choice of anaesthetic drug, consideration of unilateral treatment or changes to concurrent medication.

Burke *et al* (1987) retrospectively reviewed the charts of 136 people treated with ECT and found that complications increased with age and were also related to health status and number of medications. Similar findings have been reported by other authors (e.g. Fraser & Glass, 1978, 1980; Gaspar & Samarasinghe, 1982; Alexopoulos *et al*, 1984; Tomac *et al*, 1997). Sobin *et al* (1995) found a similar relationship between pre-existing cognitive impairment and ratings of memory impairment after treatment. Thus, for older adults, close monitoring of physical and cognitive states is recommended throughout a course of ECT. Clinic procedures will need to allow for regular routine exchange of information between the team caring for a person who is being treated with ECT and the ECT team.

Recommendations

- Age itself does not constitute a contraindication for ECT.

- People should not be denied access to ECT solely on the grounds of age.
- All coexisting medical or surgical conditions should be assessed and, where possible, stabilised or treated prior to ECT.
- The ECT clinic's treatment protocols (such as choice of anaesthetic agent) should take account of the increased likelihood of high seizure thresholds among elderly people.
- The monitoring of older people who are receiving ECT should include attention to possible changes in their physical state and cognitive function during a course of treatment.
- The ECT technique should be modified as necessary to minimise any cognitive adverse effects during ECT.

References

Alexopoulos, G. S., Shamoian, C. J., Lucas, J., et al (1984) Medical problems of geriatric psychiatric patients and younger controls during electroconvulsive therapy. *Journal of the American Geriatrics Society*, **32**, 651–654.

Benbow, S. M. (1987) The use of electroconvulsive therapy in old age psychiatry. *International Journal of Geriatric Psychiatry*, **2**, 25–30.

Benbow, S. M. (1991) Old age psychiatrists' views on the use of ECT. *International Journal of Geriatric Psychiatry*, **6**, 317–322.

Boylan, L. S., Haskett, R. F., Mulsant, B. F., et al (2000) Determinants of seizure threshold in ECT: benzodiazepine use, anesthetic dosage and other factors. *Journal of ECT*, **16**, 3–18.

Burke, W. J., Rubin, E. H., Zorumski, C. F., et al (1987) The safety of ECT in geriatric psychiatry. *Journal of the American Geriatrics Society*, **35**, 516–521.

Casey, D. A. & Davies, M. H. (1996) Electroconvulsive therapy in the very old. *General Hospital Psychiatry*, **18**, 436–439.

Cobb, A. (1995) *Older Women and ECT*. London: Mind.

Coffey, C. E., Lucke, J.. Weiner, R. D., et al (1995) Seizure threshold in electroconvulsive therapy 1: initial seizure threshold. *Biological Psychiatry*, **37**, 713–720.

Department of Health (1992) *Electroconvulsive Therapy England – Year Ending 31 March 1991*. London: Department of Health Statistics Division.

Department of Health (1999) *Electroconvulsive Therapy: Survey Covering the Period from January 1999 to March 1999, England* (Statistical Bulletin). London: Department of Health.

Department of Health (2001) *National Service Framework for Older People*. London: Department of Health.

Duffett, R., Siegert, D. R. & Lelliott, P. (1999) Electroconvulsive therapy in Wales. *Psychiatric Bulletin*, **23**, 597–601.

Fraser, R. M. & Glass, I. B. (1978) Recovery from ECT in elderly patients. *British Journal of Psychiatry*, **133**, 524–528.

Fraser, R. M. & Glass, I. B. (1980) Unilateral and bilateral ECT in elderly patients: a comparative study. *Acta Psychiatrica Scandinavica*, **62**, 13–31.

Freeman, C. (1999) Anaesthesia for electroconvulsive therapy. Statement from the Royal College of Psychiatrists' Special Committee for Electroconvulsive Therapy. *Psychiatric Bulletin*, **23**, 740–741.

Gaspar, D. & Samarasinghe, L. A. (1982) ECT in psychogeriatric practice – a sudy of risk factors, indications and outcome. *Comprehensive Psychiatry*, **23**, 170–175.

Godber, C., Rosenvinge, H., Wilkinson, D., *et al* (1987) Depression in old age: prognosis after ECT. *International Journal of Geriatric Psychiatry*, **2**, 19–24.

Karlinsky, H. & Shulman, K. T. (1984) The clinical use of electroconvulsive therapy in old age. *Journal of the American Geriatrics Society*, **32**, 183–186.

Kramer, B. A. (1987) Maintenance ECT: a survey of practice (1986). *Convulsive Therapy*, **3**, 260–268.

Olfson, M., Marcus, S., Sackeim, H. A., *et al* (1998) Use of ECT for the inpatient treatment of recurrent major depression. *American Journal of Psychiatry*, **155**, 22–29.

Pippard J. & Ellam, L. (1981) *Electroconvulsive Treatment in Great Britain, 1980*. London: Gaskell.

Prudic, J., Sackeim, H. A. & Devanand, D. P. (1990) Medication resistance and clinical response to electroconvulsive therapy. *Psychiatry Research*, **31**, 287–296.

Reid, W. H., Keller, S., Leatherman, M., *et al* (1998) ECT in Texas: 19 months of mandatory reporting. *Journal of Clinical Psychiatry*, **59**, 8–13.

Rubin, E. H., Kinscherf, D. A. & Wehrman, S. A. (1991) Response to treatment of depression in the old and the very old. *Journal of Geriatric Psychiatry and Neurology*, **4**, 65–70.

Sackeim, H. A., Decina, P., Prohovnik, I., *et al* (1987) Seizure threshold in electroconvulsive therapy: effects of sex, age, electrode placement,, and number of treatments. *Archives of General Psychiatry*, **44**, 355–360.

Sobin, C., Sackeim, H. A., Prudic, J., *et al* (1995) Predictors of retrograde amnesia following ECT. *American Journal of Psychiatry*, **152**, 995–1001.

Tomac, T. A., Rummans, T. A., Pileggi, T. S., *et al* (1997) Safety and efficacy of electroconvulsive therapy in patients over age 85. *American Journal of Geriatric Psychiatry*, **5**, 126–130.

Zervas, I. M., Calev, A., Jandorf, L., *et al* (1993) Age-dependent effects of electroconvulsive therapy on memory. *Convulsive Therapy*, **9**, 39–42.

CHAPTER 9

The use of ECT as a continuation or maintenance treatment

Richard Barnes

While ECT is effective in treating the symptoms of depression and other psychiatric conditions, relapse at the end of the course is common (Snaith, 1981; Spiker *et al*, 1985; Aronson *et al*, 1987). Usual clinical practice is for some form of prophylactic treatment – generally pharmacological single or combination therapies. However, a few patients relapse despite these methods, and such patients often require a further course of ECT in order to recover. Recently, interest has returned to the use of ECT as a prophylactic treatment in such cases (Sackeim, 1995; Rabheru & Persaud, 1997; Petrides, 1998). For a patient who has already responded to ECT, continuation treatment, if given at sufficient intervals, can reduce the overall number of treatments given in a 12-month period.

Before the advent of effective drug treatments, ECT was often used to prevent the early relapse of the index episode of illness (continuation ECT), or to prevent further episodes or recurrences of illness (maintenance ECT) (Stevenson & Geoghegan, 1951). By custom, continuation ECT has been defined as prophylactic treatment over the first 6 months of remission. Developments in pharmacotherapy have reduced its popularity, but evidence suggests it is still used quite widely (Kramer, 1987). Since it is recognised that certain patients respond only to ECT, in these cases continuation or maintenance ECT may be the treatment of choice (Loo *et al*, 1988).

The American Psychiatric Association recommended that ECT facilities offer continuation ECT as a treatment option (American Psychiatric Association, 2001).

Continuation ECT should be considered when:

- The index episode of illness responded well to ECT.
- There is early relapse despite adequate continuation drug treatment, or an inability to tolerate continuation drug treatment.
- The patient's attitude and circumstances are conducive to safe administration.

Case reports suggest prolonged courses of ECT are effective (Aronson *et al*, 1987; Theinhous *et al*, 1990) and can be given without cumulative adverse cognitive effects (Lippman *et al*, 1985; Hay & Scott, 1994; Barnes *et al*, 1997). However, there are as yet no data from a randomised controlled trial of continuation or maintenance ECT to support or refute its efficacy. This evidence gap was the major reason that the National Institute for Clinical Excellence (NICE) recommended that ECT should not be used as a long-term treatment to prevent recurrence of depressive illness (see Chapter 1). A large-scale randomised controlled trial of continuation ECT has been sponsored by the National Institute for Mental Health in the USA and this will be available when NICE reviews its guidance on ECT in November 2005.

There are likely to be some patients in the UK who will be prescribed continuation ECT. Appropriate prescription would require a proper documented assessment of the potential risks and benefits of treatment, for which valid informed consent had been obtained. At least patients who are to consider continuation treatment will have the personal experience to trade off the potential benefits and adverse effects of treatment. Evidence-based guidelines for continuation ECT are not available, but up-to-date citations of the relevant clinical evidence are available in American Psychiatric Association (2001) and Andrade & Kurinji (2002). An example of a protocol from one ECT clinic is given in Appendix IX to promote discussion of best practice.

References

American Psychiatric Association (2001) *The Practice of Electroconvulsive Therapy: Recommendations for Treatment, Training and Privileging* (2nd edn). Washington, DC: APA.

Andrade, C. & Kurinji, S. (2002) Continuation and maintenance ECT: a review of recent research. *Journal of ECT*, **18**, 149–158.

Aronson, A. A., Shukla, S. & Hoff, A. (1987) Continuation therapy after ECT for delusional depression. A naturalistic study of prophylactic treatments for relapse. *Convulsive Therapy*, **3**, 251–259.

Barnes, R. C., Hussein, A., Anderson, D. N., *et al* (1997) Maintenance electroconvulsive therapy and cognitive function. *British Journal of Psychiatry*, **170**, 285–287.

Hay, A. G. & Scott, A. I. (1994) Electroconvulsive therapy and brain damage (letter). *British Journal of Psychiatry*, **165**, 120–121.

Kramer, B. A. (1987) Maintenance ECT: a survey of practice (1986). *Convulsive Therapy*, **3**, 260–268.

Lippman, S., Manshadi, M., Wehry, M., *et al* (1985) 1,250 electroconvulsive treatments without evidence of brain injury. *British Journal of Psychiatry*, **147**, 203–204.

Loo, H., Galinowski, A., Boccara, I., *et al* (1988) Benefit of maintenance ECT in recurrent depression. *L'Encephale*, **14**, 39–41.

Monroe, R. R. (1991) Maintenance electroconvulsive therapy. *Psychiatric Clinics of North America*, **14**, 947–960.

Petrides, G. (1998) Continuation ECT: a review. *Psychiatric Annals*, **28**, 517–523.

Rabheru, K. & Persaud, E. (1997) A review of continuation and maintenance electroconvulsive therapy. *Canadian Journal of Psychiatry*, **42**, 476–484.

Sackeim, H. A. (1995) Continuation therapy following ECT: directions for future research. *Psychopharmacology Bulletin*, **30**, 501–531.

Snaith, R. P. (1981) How much ECT does the depressed patient need? In *Electroconvulsive Therapy: An Appraisal* (ed. R. L. Palmer), pp. 61–64. New York: Oxford University Press.

Spiker, D. G., Stein, J. & Rich, C. L. (1985) Delusional depression and electroconvulsive therapy: one year later. *Convulsive Therapy*, **1**, 167–172.

Stevenson, G. H. & Geoghegan, J. J. (1951) Prophylactic electroshock. *American Journal of Psychiatry*, **107**, 743–748.

Theinhous, O. J., Margletta, S. & Bennett, J. A. (1990) A study of the clinical efficacy of maintenance ECT. *Journal of Clinical Psychiatry*, **51**, 141–144.

Part II
Psychotropic drug treatment and ECT

Systematic review of psychotropic medication given during a course of ECT for depressive illness: therapeutic and adverse consequences

Andrew M. McIntosh and Stephen M. Lawrie

Introduction

Before administering ECT a patient's current medication and its likely effect on the action of ECT is usually considered. Medication for general medical conditions is usually continued, but the correct strategy regarding psychotropic medication is somewhat less clear to clinicians. The guidelines provided by the American Psychiatric Association (2001) conflict with the advice given in the first edition of the present book. The practice of continuing some medications (e.g. lithium or anti-depressants) is generally based on the possibility of a synergistic effect with the response to ECT, while patients are exposed to minimal additional risk. The strategy of discontinuing benzodiazepines is based on their tendency to inhibit seizures and consequently the clinical effect of ECT.

The uncertainty about which medications can be safely continued during ECT may be due to several factors. First, current guidelines are heavily influenced by expert opinion. Second, to our knowledge, no systematic review of concurrent medication and ECT has been per-formed. Finally, the evidence quoted in guidelines is generally from observational studies, which are more prone to bias than randomised controlled trials (RCTs).

This chapter systematically reviews the evidence for the therapeutic and adverse effects of psychotropic medication administered during a course of ECT. Evidence from RCTs is used wherever possible. Data on adverse and therapeutic effects occurring during or immediately after ECT are considered in the first instance and, when appropriate, combined using meta-analysis. Where long-term data exist for patients randomised to an active drug versus a comparator, this is presented in the text.

Methods

We conducted a systematic review of RCTs that compared patients treated with ECT and a concomitant psychotropic medication with either ECT alone, ECT and placebo or ECT and another psychotropic medication.

Search strategy

We searched Medline, Embase and PsychINFO through the Ovid interface, and the Cochrane Register of Clinical Trials through the Update-Software website. The strategy included the search terms 'ECT', 'drug therapy' and related terms, both as expanded subject headings and as free text (the exact details of the search strategy are available from the authors on request). A thesaurus or MeSH browser was used to identify the related terms. Search results were exported directly to Reference Manager software and any duplicates were removed. The search results were inspected by both reviewers independently, with disagreements being resolved by discussion. The reference lists of included articles were also inspected for further studies.

Information from individual studies is abstracted below in tabular form according to the following headings: inclusion/exclusion criteria, intervention(s), quality, number of subjects, number lost to follow-up, length of follow-up and outcome measure(s). The column 'quality' summarises information allocation concealment, blinding and the use of intention-to-treat analysis (all studies were randomised). The results of each trial are summarised and used in the subsequent meta-analysis when two or more trials considered the same interventions.

Definition of treatment with psychotropic medication

Initially we intended to consider only pharmacological interventions prescribed as antidepressants, mood stabilisers or antipsychotics. However, many interventions were difficult to classify (e.g. calcium antagonists and pindolol). We therefore decided to consider any pharmacological intervention, with the exception of anaesthetic gases.

Meta-analysis

The primary measure of treatment efficacy used was 'mean rating scale improvement'. For adverse events we considered the dichotomous outcome 'leaving the study for any reason' as an index of tolerability and also the 'total number of side-effects' as a continuous measure. *Post hoc* analyses were also conducted on the basis of the data available. Continuous data were combined to produce pooled estimates of standardised difference and event-like data were pooled to produce combined estimates of relative risk. Analyses were based on intention to treat whenever this was available, and completer-only analysis when it was not. Between-study heterogeneity was investigated using a χ^2 analysis and where this was significant we present both the fixed- and random-effects estimates of treatment effect. Otherwise fixed-effect analyses only are presented. We did not anticipate having sufficient data to make any planned subgroup comparisons or sensitivity analyses.

Results

A total of 644 references were located from the four biomedical databases. The distribution of abstracts according to database is shown in Table 10.1. Of the 240 articles that were retrieved in full, 40 belonged to one of the pre-specified study types. No systematic reviews and 17 trials were identified. The results are presented below according to study type.

ECT and antidepressants versus ECT alone, or ECT and placebo

Four trials compared the effects of ECT and an antidepressant with those of ECT and placebo (Seager & Bird, 1962; Imlah *et al*, 1965; Lauritzen *et al*, 1996; Mayur *et al*, 2000).

In the first and oldest study, Seager & Bird (1962) randomised 19 patients to imipramine and 21 patients to placebo. After a week of receiving medication ECT was commenced. All patients responded satisfactorily to ECT, although slightly fewer treatments were given to those receiving imipramine than to those receiving placebo (6.3 compared with 7). Adverse effects were not reported in the trial and it is not clear if they were measured.

Table 10.1 Distribution of abstracts according to database

Database	Number of randomised controlled trials identified
Medline	371
Embase	312
PsychINFO	55
Cochrane Register of Clinical Trials	263
Total references (duplicates removed)	644

Imlah *et al* (1965) randomised 150 patients to ECT plus phenelzine, ECT plus imipramine or ECT plus placebo in equal proportions. ECT was discontinued after two raters agreed that a patient had reached a maximal response. The average number of ECT treatments given to each group was slightly higher in the placebo-treated patients (7.9 compared with 6.9 with phenelzine and 7.1 with imipramine), although the differences were not said to be significant. Standard deviations were not reported. Adverse effects were not reported in the trial and it is not clear if they were measured.

Lauritzen *et al* (1996) randomised patients with electrocardiographic (ECG) impairment to either ECT and paroxetine or ECT and placebo. Eighteen patients received ECT and paroxetine, and 17 received ECT and placebo. Similar numbers of ECT treatments were received by the two groups (12.1 and 11.1, respectively) and the duration of seizures in both groups was also similar. Immediately after the final ECT treatment, the mean score on the Hamilton Rating Scale for Depression (HRSD) was 8.9 (s.d.=4.7) in the paroxetine-treated group and 9.2 (s.d.=3.4) in the placebo-treated group. Two patients were withdrawn, both from the paroxetine group, one because of side-effects (stomach pains), the other for a lack of therapeutic response.

Mayur *et al* (2000), using an antidepressant discontinuation design, randomised 15 patients with DSM–IV major depression to ECT and continued antidepressant treatment and 15 to treatment with ECT and placebo (antidepressant discontinuation). No significant differences were observed in terms of speed of response to ECT, although the ECT plus antidepressant-treated group had higher ratings on an anticholinergic side-effects rating scale.

ECT and an antidepressant versus ECT and another antidepressant

The results of the study by Imlah *et al* (1965), in which 100 patients received either ECT plus phenelzine or ECT plus imipramine, are described above. In that study, patients were followed up at 6 months and the proportion of people remaining well was 78% in both antidepressant groups.

In a second part to their study, Lauritzen *et al* (1996) randomised people *without* ECG impairment to receive either paroxetine (27) or imipramine (25). The mean number of ECT treatments was similar: 11.1 for patients on paroxetine and 10.2 for those on imipramine. Three patients randomised to imipramine were withdrawn, two because of side-effects. Four subjects were withdrawn in the paroxetine group, though in only one patient was this probably due to an adverse event. At the end of ECT, patients treated with imipramine had lower HRSD scores and lower melancholia scores than those treated with paroxetine.

Bernardo et al (2000) included 18 subjects in their 'pilot' study, which randomised people meeting DSM–IV criteria for major depressive episode to either ECT and concurrent venlafaxine (9) or ECT and either concurrent clomipramine or imipramine (9). The number of ECT treatments, the mean seizure duration and the average increases in blood pressure after ECT did not differ significantly between the two groups.

ECT and lithium versus ECT alone or ECT and placebo

A single trial comparing concurrent ECT plus lithium and concurrent ECT plus placebo was found, in which 38 patients participated (Coppen et al, 1981). Lithium and placebo were begun during ECT, although it is not clear at which point this took place. Five people in the placebo arm failed to respond to an initial course of ECT, compared with only two in the lithium arm.

Calcium antagonists

One study compared ECT and nicardipine with ECT and placebo (Dubovsky et al, 2001). Twenty-six patients with depression that met DSM–IV criteria were randomised and compared in terms of their mean scores on the HRSD, the Mini-Mental State Examination (MMSE) and several tests of cognition. No differences were found in terms of number of ECT treatments or mean total seizure duration. Nicardipine-treated patients improved more than placebo-treated patients. No differences were found in MMSE scores.

Concurrent treatment with synthetic hormones

Three trials examined the effects of exogenous hormone administration on ECT (Feighner et al, 1972; Mattes et al, 1989, 1990; Stern et al, 1991).

Feighner et al (1972) compared the effects on ECT of concurrent dexamethasone treatment with placebo. The number of ECT treatments received was greater in the dexamethasone-treated patients than in those treated with placebo and the mean time to maximum improvement was longer in those treated with dexamethasone. After 22 days of treatment, dexamethasone-treated patients did non-significantly worse than placebo-treated patients on one outcome measure (Zung scale, a composite scale which included items from the HRSD and Renard scale).

The second trial (Mattes et al, 1989, 1990) compared concurrent vasopressin treatment with that of placebo. Thirty-three patients were randomised to the two groups. No significant differences were found between the groups on several cognitive measures, though the results tended to favour vasopressin-treated subjects. Improvement in depression was also similar between the two groups, though the vasopressin-treated patients had somewhat higher post-ECT HRSD scores (11.07 compared with 9.57).

A third trial, involving a total of 20 patients and described as preliminary, compared concomitant ECT and the thyroid hormone T3 with ECT and placebo (Stern *et al*, 1991). T3-treated patients required significantly fewer ECT treatments than placebo-treated patients (8.0 compared with 12.2) and a greater proportion achieved a higher antidepressant response. The cognitive adverse effects of ECT differed significantly for the outcome 'recall of personal events', with T3-treated patients recalling more personal events. Other cognitive effects did not differ between the groups, though they tended to favour T3-treated patients.

Treatment with tryptophan

Two trials have examined the effects of tryptophan on ECT in controlled trials (d'Elia *et al*, 1977, 1978; Kirkegaard *et al*, 1978).

Kirkegaard *et al* (1978) randomised 20 patients to either ECT and intravenous tryptophan or ECT and intravenous placebo (saline) in equal numbers. HRSD ratings were made before the first application of ECT and after the final time. The mean number of treatments given to the tryptophan group was 9.5 (s.d.=3.9) compared with 10.5 (s.d.=2.6) in the placebo group. This difference was not significant. Similarly, no differences were found in mean HRSD scores at end-point.

A further trial was found in which patients were randomised to either ECT and tryptophan or ECT and placebo (d'Elia *et al*, 1977, 1978). Depression was rated using a number of measures, including the Zung rating scale and a 15-point rating scale of depression, although only a subsample were asked to rate adverse effects. Four days after the final ECT treatment, no differences were found between the groups in terms of either adverse effects or clinician's global rating. Tryptophan-treated patients required slightly fewer ECT treatments and had slightly better HRSD scores at day 16 of the trial, but neither difference was statistically significant. Overall, there were no significant differences in adverse effects.

Other strategies

Kay *et al* (1970) compared the effects of concurrent amitriptyline or diazepam administered during ECT and continued afterwards. More patients in the amitriptyline-treated arm ceased to take medication because of side-effects (6 of the 59 on amitriptyline compared with 1 of 73 on diazepam). However, three patients, all in the diazepam group, committed suicide and the therapeutic effects favoured amitriptyline patients overall.

Arfwidsson *et al* (1973) randomised in-patients with endogenous depression to ECT and concurrent chlorpromazine (50–150 mg) or to ECT and concurrent placebo. No significant differences were found in terms of either recovery from depression or the duration of seizures.

Rosenquist *et al* (1994) performed a crossover trial in which patients were randomised before a course of ECT to either caffeine benzoate or placebo. Patients were then given the treatment they had not previously received. Caffeine before treatment had no effect on three measures of seizure activity or on four measures of heart rate.

Shiah *et al* (2000) randomised 20 patients with depressive disorder to receive either pindolol (9) or placebo (11) during a course of ECT. One patient dropped out of the pindolol arm of the study and four dropped out of the placebo arm. Therapeutic measures favoured the pindolol-treated patients, however. Significantly more patients in the pindolol arm improved during the course of six ECT treatments than in the placebo-treated group. Mean HRSD scores were also significantly lower in the pindolol-treated patients.

Sachs *et al* (1989) randomly assigned 11 patients to either placebo (6) or ergoloid salicylates (containing hydergine, a drug sometimes used to treat dementia). One patient in the placebo arm dropped out. Most memory measures deteriorated in both groups over time. Only one memory measure, delayed recall, was found to improve more in the ergoloid-treated patients than in those treated with placebo. The reduction in HRSD score was also significantly greater in ergoloid-treated patients than in placebo-treated patients.

Meta-analysis

Antidepressants versus placebo

Three trials provided rating scale data at the end of the course of ECT. However, standard deviations were not reported in two of these. Data from the one remaining trial showed no significant difference between placebo and antidepressants, though the antidepressant-treated patients had slightly lower scores overall (SES = –0.07, 95% CI –0.74 to 0.59). The same trial also showed no significant difference between the groups in terms of the number of ECT treatments received (SES = 0.19, 95% CI –0.48 to 0.85).

The three trials of antidepressants provided data for the outcome 'drop-out for any reason'. No significant difference in drop-out was found in either direction (relative risk = 0.97, 95% CI 0.84 to 1.1) (Figure 10.1).

Tryptophan versus placebo

For the outcome 'drop-out for any reason', both trials provided data. Some event rates in the placebo arm were zero and relative risks could

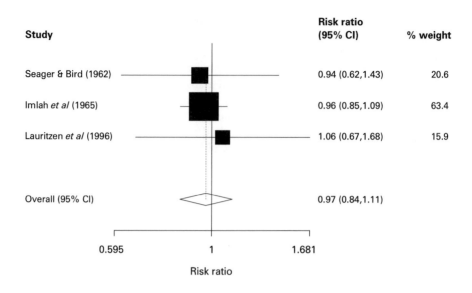

Figure 10.1 Meta-analysis of antidepressants versus placebo for the outcome 'drop-out for any reason'. Summary measure shown is relative risk, created using STATA 7.

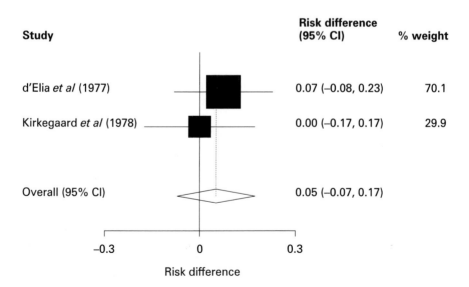

Figure 10.2 Meta-analysis of tryptophan versus placebo for the outcome 'drop-out for any reason'. Summary measure shown is risk difference.

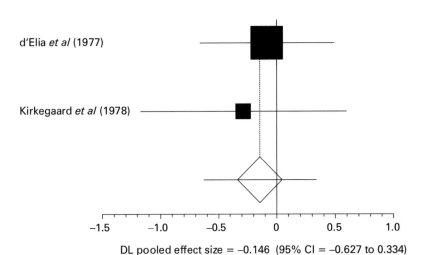

Effect size meta-analysis plot (random effects)

DL pooled effect size = –0.146 (95% CI = –0.627 to 0.334)

Figure 10.3 Meta-analysis of tryptophan versus placebo for the outcome 'mean numbers of ECT treatments received'. Summary measure is standardised effect size. DL, DerSimonian–Laird estimation of heterogeneity.

not be used for meta-analysis. Risk differences were therefore combined to produce a summary measure of effect size. No difference in drop-out was found between patients treated with concurrent tryptophan or placebo during ECT (risk difference = 0.05, 95% CI –0.07 to 0.17) (Figure 10.2). Similarly, no differences were found between the groups in terms of the number of ECT treatments received by patients (SES = –0.15, 95% CI –0.63 to 0.33) (Figure 10.3). Neither trial provided sufficient data to calculate a summary measure of rating scale improvement.

Discussion

Seventeen randomised controlled trials were found that had compared pharmacotherapy with either placebo or another drug. All interventions were given during a course of ECT. Most studies concerned antidepressants, though lithium, pindolol, tryptophan, vasopressin, ergoloids and T3 were all represented in at least one trial. The best available evidence was for the efficacy of antidepressants compared with placebo. Other trials also showed T3, lithium, lithium augmentation of antidepressant drugs and pindolol to be more effective in terms of clinical improvement. Trials comparing tryptophan, vasopressin and ergoloids with placebo were more equivocal.

Table 10.2 Summary of the methods of the randomised controlled trials included in the systematic review

Trial	Inclusion/ exclusion criteria	Intervention(s)	Quality	Number of subjects	Loss to follow-up	Length of follow-up	Outcome measure(s)
Arfwidsson et al (1973)	In-patients < 65 years with 'endogenous' or 'endogenous-psychogenic' depression	ECT + chlorpromazine; ECT + placebo	AC: unclear; double blind; ITT: no	57	14	Up to 72 days	'Recovery', number of treatments and 'days in hospital'
Bernardo et al (2000)	DSM–IV major depressive episode; HRSD ≥ 18	ECT + venlafaxine (150 mg); ECT + tricyclic antidepressant	AC: unclear; raters blind; ITT: no	18	None reported	Until HRSD ≤ 7	Number of treatments; seizure duration; increase in blood pressure
Coppen et al (1981)	Research Diagnostic Criteria; HRSD score ≥ 16 before ECT	ECT + lithium carbonate; ECT + placebo	AC: unclear; double blind; ITT: no	38	Unclear	52 weeks	Mean HRSD score at 52 weeks
d'Elia et al (1977, 1978)	Patients < 65 years with endogenous depressive syndromes	ECT + tryptophan; ECT + placebo	AC: unclear; double blind; ITT: no	47	12	1 month	Zung rating scale, duration of seizure, drop-out, memory function
Dubovsky et al (2001)	In-patients with DSM–IV major depressive disorder	ECT + nicardipine; ECT + placebo	AC: unclear; double blind; ITT: no	26	Unclear	6 months	Numerous depression and memory scales
Feighner et al (1972)	In-patients with primary depression	ECT + placebo; ECT + dexamethasone	AC: unclear; double blind; ITT: no	18	Unclear	Up to 22 days	Zung rating scale, 'symptom remission'

Study	Patients	Intervention	Methodology	n	Drop-out	Follow-up	Outcome measures
Imlah et al (1965)	In-patients with depressive illness	ECT + phenelzine; ECT + imipramine; ECT + placebo	AC: unclear; only patients blinded; ITT: no	150	39	6 months	'Remained well' (undefined)
Kay et al (1970)	'Affective disorders' uncomplicated by schizophrenia, organic brain disease or 'subnormality'	ECT + amitriptyline (50–150 mg); ECT + diazepam (4–12 mg)	AC: unclear; double blind; ITT, no	132	17 or more (unclear)	7 months	'Unsatisfactory progress', drop-out, mean HRSD score
Kirkegaard et al (1978)	Patients with endogenous depression	ECT + placebo; ECT + tryptophan	AC: unclear; double blind; ITT: no	20	0	Unclear	HRSD score
Lauritzen et al (1996)	DSM-III-R major depressive episode; ECT responders (HRSD score < 13)	ECT + paroxetine vs ECT + placebo for people with ECG impairment (group A); ECT + imipramine (100–300 mg) vs ECT + paroxetine (20–60 mg) for people without ECG impairment (group B)	AC: unclear; double blind; ITT: no	Group A, 35; group B, 52	Group A, 7; group B, 8	6 months	Proportion remaining well at 6 months; time to relapse (relapse defined as HRSD score ≥ 18, MES score ≥ 15 on two occasions)
Mattes et al (1989, 1990)	DSM-III major depressive disorder	ECT + vasopressin; ECT + placebo	AC: unclear; double blind; ITT: no	33	Unclear	48 hours following final ECT	HRSD score and numerous memory measures
Mayur et al (2000)	DSM-IV major depression treated with antidepressants	ECT + placebo; ECT + continuation antidepressants	AC: unclear; investigators and patients blinded; ITT: no	30	8	42 days	MADRS and HRSD scores

Table continues over

95

Table 10.2 *Continued*

Trial	Inclusion/ exclusion criteria	Intervention(s)	Quality	Number of subjects	Loss to follow-up	Length of follow-up	Outcome measure(s)
Rosenquist et al (1994)	Major depression	ECT + caffeine pre-treatment; ECT + placebo	Crossover; AC: unclear; investigators and patients blinded; ITT: unclear	12	Unclear	Until end of ECT course	EEG measures and heart rate
Sachs et al (1989)	Patients to be treated with ECT	ECT + ergoloid mesylates; ECT + placebo	AC: unclear; patients/raters blinded; ITT: no	11	1	After 2 treatments	Memory, HRSD score
Seager & Bird (1962)	In-patients with moderate–severe depressive illness with retardation/agitation and pessimism	ECT + imipramine; ECT + placebo	AC: unclear; clinicians blind; ITT: no	40	15	6 months	Relapse (undefined)
Shiah et al (2000)	DSM–IV major depressive disorder	ECT + pindolol; ECT + placebo	AC: unclear; double-blind; ITT: no	20	5	Until end of HRSD course	HRSD score
Stern et al (1991)	DSM–III–R major depression, comorbid axis I disorders excluded	ECT + T3; ECT + placebo	AC: unclear; double blind; ITT: no	20	Unclear	Until end of course	HRSD score

AC, allocation concealment; ITT, intention-to-treat analysis (yes/no); MADRS, Montgomery–Asberg Depression Rating Scale; MES, Melancholia Scale.

Unfortunately, most trials either did not report adverse effects or did not consider them. This is regrettable as the decision to co-prescribe drugs and ECT is likely to focus on safety issues, particularly those occurring during ECT administration. Cognition was considered by some studies, though the results were generally equivocal. Three suicides occurred in a single trial of diazepam versus amitriptyline. Although too few patients were randomised to rule out a chance finding, the greater number of suicides in the diazepam arm might reflect an inhibitory effect of diazepam on the efficacy of ECT.

Most trials randomised patients to drugs that were begun before ECT was started. In others, however, the timing of administration was less clear. Many studies reported long-term side-effects occurring after the end of ECT. In these studies, patients were generally taking the drugs to which they were originally randomised. Therefore, long-term therapeutic effects may be due to their efficacy at maintaining remission rather than any synergistic effect with ECT.

Overall, the lack of large trials or common outcome measures between studies severely limits the interpretation of the available evidence. That which is available suggests that therapeutic responses to ECT may be augmented by antidepressants, lithium and pindolol without any major risks to patients. There is a clear need for pragmatic RCTs of pharmacological interventions given during a course of electroconvulsive therapy.

References

American Psychiatric Association (2001) *The Practice of Electroconvulsive Therapy: Recommendations for Treatment, Training and Privileging.* Washington, DC: APA.

Arfwidsson, L., Arn, L., Beskow, J., *et al* (1973) Chlorpromazine and the anti-depressive efficacy of electroconvulsive therapy. *Acta Psychiatrica Scandinavica*, **49**, 580–587.

Bernardo, M., Navarro, V., Salva, J., *et al* (2000) Seizure activity and safety in combined treatment with venlafaxine and ECT: a pilot study. *Journal of ECT*, **16**, 38–42.

Coppen, A., Abou-Saleh, M. T., Milln, P., *et al* (1981) Lithium continuation therapy following electroconvulsive therapy. *British Journal of Psychiatry*, **139**, 284–287.

d'Elia, G., Lehmann, J. & Raotma, H. (1977) Evaluation of the combination of tryptophan and ECT in the treatment of depression. I. Clinical analysis. *Acta Psychiatrica Scandinavica*, **56**, 303–318.

d'Elia, G., Lehmann, J. & Raotma, H. (1978) Influence of tryptophan on memory functions in depressive patients treated with unilateral ECT. *Acta Psychiatrica Scandinavica*, **57**, 259–268.

Dubovsky, S. L., Buzan, R., Thomas, M., *et al* (2001) Nicardipine improves the antidepressant action of ECT but does not improve cognition. *Journal of ECT*, **17**, 3–10.

Feighner, J. P., King, L. J., Schuckit, M. A., *et al* (1972) Hormonal potentiation of imipramine and ECT in primary depression. *American Journal of Psychiatry*, **128**, 1230–1238.

Imlah, N. W., Ryan, E. & Harrington, J. A. (1965) The influence of antidepressant drugs on the response to electroconvulsive therapy and on subsequent relapse rates. *Neuropsychopharmacology*, **4**, 438–442.

Kay, D. W., Fahy, T. & Garside, R. F. (1970) A seven-month double-blind trial of amitriptyline and diazepam in ECT-treated depressed patients. *British Journal of Psychiatry*, **117**, 667–671.

Kirkegaard, C., Moller, S. E. & Bjorum, N. (1978) Addition of L-tryptophan to electroconvulsive treatment in endogenous depression. A double-blind study. *Acta Psychiatrica Scandinavica*, **58**, 457–462.

Lauritzen, L., Odgaard, K., Clemmesen, L., *et al* (1996) Relapse prevention by means of paroxetine in ECT-treated patients with major depression: a comparison with imipramine and placebo in medium-term continuation therapy. *Acta Psychiatrica Scandinavica*, **94**, 241–251.

Mattes, J. A., Pettinati, H. M., Nilsen, S. M., *et al* (1989) Vasopressin for ECT-induced memory impairment: a placebo-controlled comparison. *Psychopharmacology Bulletin*, **25**, 80–84.

Mattes, J. A., Pettinati, H. M., Stephens, S., *et al* (1990) A placebo-controlled evaluation of vasopressin for ECT-induced memory impairment. *Biological Psychiatry*, **27**, 289–303.

Mayur, P. M., Gangadhar, B. N., Subbakrishna, D. K., *et al* (2000) Discontinuation of antidepressant drugs during electroconvulsive therapy: a controlled study. *Journal of Affective Disorders*, **58**, 37–41.

Rosenquist, P. B., McCall, W. V., Farah, A., *et al* (1994) Effects of caffeine pretreatment on measures of seizure impact. *Convulsive Therapy*, **10**, 181–185.

Sachs, G. S., Gelenberg, A. J., Bellinghausen, B., *et al* (1989) Ergoloid mesylates and ECT. *Journal of Clinical Psychiatry*, **50**, 87–90.

Seager, C. P. & Bird, R. L. (1962) Imipramine with electrical treatment in depression – a controlled trial. *Journal of Mental Science*, **108**, 704–707.

Shiah, I. S., Yatham, L. N., Srisurapanont, M., *et al* (2000) Does the addition of pindolol accelerate the response to electroconvulsive therapy in patients with major depression? A double-blind, placebo-controlled pilot study. *Journal of Clinical Psychopharmacology*, **20**, 373–378.

Stern, R. A., Nevels, C. T., Shelhorse, M. E., *et al* (1991) Antidepressant and memory effects of combined thyroid hormone treatment and electroconvulsive therapy: preliminary findings. *Biological Psychiatry*, **30**, 623–627.

CHAPTER 11

Systematic review. Continuation pharmacotherapy after ECT for depressive illness

Andrew M. Mcintosh and Stephen M. Lawrie

Introduction

Electroconvulsive therapy (ECT) is commonly administered to patients with severe and medication-resistant depressive illness. Although the initial response rate is high, the relapse rate 1 year after successful treatment probably exceeds only 50% (O'Leary & Lee, 1996). In an attempt to reduce the relapse rate, continuation pharmacotherapy is usually prescribed once remission has been achieved. Although some trials have been conducted, there are no systematic overviews of treatments to guide clinical practice.

This chapter systematically reviews the randomised evidence for continuation pharmacotherapy following a successful course of ECT.

Methods

We conducted a systematic review of randomised controlled trials (RCTs) that had compared the efficacy of pharmacotherapy with placebo, another pharmacological intervention or continuation ECT. The search strategy was as set out for the systematic review in Chapter 10, and the results are similarly presented below. In brief, we searched Medline, Embase, PsychINFO and the Cochrane Register of Clinical Trials databases for the search terms 'ECT', 'drug therapy' and related terms. The reference lists of retrieved articles were inspected for further studies. The results of each trial are summarised below and are used in the subsequent meta-analysis when two or more trials considered the same interventions. In the meta-analysis, data have been combined to produce pooled estimates of relative risk. Analyses have been based on intention-to-treat analysis whenever this was available, and completer-only analysis when it was not. Between-study heterogeneity was investigated using a χ^2 analysis and where this was significant we present both the fixed- and random-effects estimates of treatment effect. Otherwise fixed-effect analyses only are presented. We did not anticipate having sufficient data to make any planned subgroup comparisons or sensitivity analyses.

Results

A total of 870 references were located from the four biomedical databases (see Chapter 10 and Table 10.1). Of the 240 articles retrieved in full, 40 belonged to one of the pre-specified study types. Six relevant RCTs were identified from the initial search and three more were obtained from the inspection of reference lists. The results according to study type are shown below. Of the nine RCTs identified (Table 11.1), five considered the efficacy of antidepressants against placebo, two against an alternative antidepressant and one against tricyclic augmentation with lithium. Two trials concerned melatonin augmentation of a selective serotonin reuptake inhibitor (SSRI) (one RCT), lithium augmentation of a tricyclic antidepressant (one RCT) or lithium therapy alone (one RCT). One study considered augmentation of antidepressant therapy in patients with psychotic depression (Meyers et al, 2001). The trials were methodologically heterogeneous. Only three had randomised patients once remission had been established with ECT (Grunhaus et al, 2001; Meyers et al, 2001; Sackeim et al, 2001). The remaining trials all administered antidepressants during the ECT treatment phase. In all cases it was difficult to ascertain which method of randomisation had been used and whether there had been adequate allocation concealment.

Antidepressants versus placebo or other antidepressants

Five RCTs considered the efficacy of antidepressants against that of placebo (Seager & Bird, 1962; Imlah et al, 1965; Krog-Meyer et al, 1984; Lauritzen et al, 1996; Sackeim et al, 2001).

Seager & Bird (1962) randomised 43 patients with moderate–severe depression (undefined) to receive either imipramine or placebo for 1 week before their course of ECT began. Patients responding to ECT who continued in the trial were then randomised a second time to receive either imipramine or placebo. It is not clear from the methods whether only a proportion were re-randomised or by what method randomisation was accomplished. Patients were then followed up for a maximum of 6 months or until relapse. Of the 28 people for whom data were available, 2 of 12 relapsed in the imipramine group compared with 11 of 16 in the placebo group ($\chi^2 = 5.5$, $P = 0.019$).

Imlah et al (1965) randomised 150 in-patients with 'depression of a sufficient degree to warrant the use of ECT' to ECT plus phenelzine, ECT plus imipramine or ECT plus placebo. All tablets were given three times daily (including placebo) but it is not clear how patients were randomised or how the allocation was concealed. Patients were randomised to each therapy at the start of ECT, and if a clinical response was observed to ECT, medication was continued for a further 3 months and the proportion of patients in each group relapsing was compared. The trial found that more patients receiving antidepressants remained well at 6 months compared with those receiving placebo ($\chi^2 = 11.9$, $P < 0.01$). The proportion of people remaining well in the two antidepressant groups was equal, however.

Krog-Meyer et al (1984) randomised patients with depression that both met ICD–8 criteria and were predicted to relapse, on the basis of a test of thyrotrophin-releasing hormone (TRH), to either amitriptyline ($n = 11$) or placebo ($n = 13$). The primary outcome measure was relapse, defined as an increase in the dose of antidepressant or placebo, or a change to another antidepressant. Median scores on the Hamilton Rating Scale for Depression (HRSD) were also compared between groups, although significance tests were not conducted. Two patients randomised to amitriptyline relapsed compared with nine of those randomised to placebo.

Lauritzen et al (1996) selected two groups of patients, patients with electrocardiogram (ECG) abnormality and those without. Those with ECG abnormality were randomised to paroxetine or placebo during treatment with ECT and those without were all randomised to either imipramine or paroxetine. Those patients failing to achieve remission with ECT were withdrawn from the study. Seventy-four patients were included in the 6-month continuation phase and were followed up for a total of 6 months. In the group with ECG abnormalities, 15 patients received paroxetine and 16 received placebo. In the group with normal ECGs, 21 patients received paroxetine (mean dose 28.5 mg) and 22 received imipramine (mean dose 138 mg). A number of people left the trial prematurely (see Table 11.1). In the group with ECG abnormalities, after 3 months patients receiving paroxetine were significantly more likely to remain well than those receiving placebo, although at 6 months this difference had become non-significant. In the goup with normal ECGs, patients receiving paroxetine were more likely to remain well at 3 months and at end-point than those receiving imipramine ($P \leq 0.05$).

Sackeim et al (2001) randomised patients to receive either nortriptyline ($n = 27$) or placebo ($n = 29$) for up to 24 weeks. The main outcome measures were 'relapse of major depressive disorder' as a proportion of the group randomised and 'time to relapse' using the Kaplan–Maier method. The relapse rate for placebo-treated patients was 84% (95% CI 70–99) compared with 60% (95% CI 41–79) for those treated with nortriptyline. This trend was also evident on non-parametric survival analysis.

Table 11.1 Included randomised controlled trials

Trial	Inclusion/ exclusion criteria	Intervention(s)	Quality	Number of subjects	Loss to follow-up	Length of follow-up	Outcome measure(s)
Coppen et al (1981)	Research Diagnostic Criteria; HRSD score ≥ 16 before ECT	Lithium carbonate/placebo started during ECT phase; patients were begun on treatment during ECT and could receive other treatments during the trial	AC: unclear; double blind; ITT: no	38	Unclear	52 weeks	Mean HRSD score at 52 weeks
Grunhaus et al (2001)	DSM–IV major depressive disorder; post ECT HRSD ≤ 10	Fluoxetine (30–40 mg); fluoxetine (30–40 mg) + melatonin (5 or 10 mg)	AC: unclear; double blind; ITT: no	35	4	3 months	Relapse (≥ DSM–IV symptoms); HRSD ≥ 16
Imlah et al (1965)	In-patients with depressive illness	Phenelzine; imipramine; placebo. Patients were begun on drug during ECT	AC: unclear; only patients blinded; ITT: no	150	39	6 months	'Remained well' (undefined)
Kay et al (1970)	'Affective disorders' uncomplicated by schizophrenia, organic brain disease or 'subnormality'	Amitriptyline (50–150 mg); diazepam (4–12 mg). Patients were begun on drug during ECT and could receive other treatments during the trial	AC: unclear; double blind; ITT, no	132	17 or more (unclear)	7 months	'Relapse', 'unsatisfactory progress', overdose after 1 month of drug treatment
Krog-Meyer et al (1984)	ICD–8 depression; only patients predicted to relapse on the basis of a TRH test were randomised	Amitriptyline or placebo; patients could be taken out of one group and transferred to another	AC: unclear; psychiatrist; blind; ITT: no; unequal treatment?	24	Unclear	Study continued for 6 months	Relapse (defined as an increase in antidepressant dose or change to another class of antidepressant

Study	Diagnosis	Intervention	Methods			Duration	Outcome
Lauritzen et al (1996)	DSM-III-R major depressive episode; ECT responders (HRSD score < 13)	Group A: paroxetine vs placebo for people with ECG impairment; group B: imipramine (100–300 mg) vs paroxetine (20–60 mg) for people without ECG impairment; patients were begun on treatment during ECT and could receive other treatments during the trial. All patients started on treatment initially and were either randomised to continue or to change to another drug/placebo	AC: unclear; double blind; ITT: no	Group A, 31; group B, 43	Group A, 7; group B, 8	6 months	Proportion remaining well at 6 months; time to relapse (relapse defined as HRSD score $\geq$ 18, MES score $\geq$ 15 on two occasions)
Meyers et al (2001)	DSM-IV unipolar psychotic major depression + HRSD <10 after ECT	Nortriptyline and placebo; nortriptyline and perphenazine	AC: unclear; patients blind; ITT: no	28	Unclear	26 weeks	Relapse (DSM-IV major depression, delusional ideation)
Sackeim et al (2001)	RDC; HRSD score reduced 60% by ECT. Exclusions: bipolar disorder, schizophrenia, alcohol/drug misuse and ECT in last 6 months	Nortriptyline; nortriptyline and lithium; placebo	AC: unclear; double blind; ITT: no	84	11	24 weeks	Time to 'relapse' (defined as HRSD $\geq$ 16)
Seager & Bird (1962)	In-patients with moderate–severe depressive illness with retardation/agitation and pessimism	Imipramine; placebo. Patients were begun on drug treatment during ECT	AC: unclear; clinicians blind; ITT: no	43	15	6 months	Relapse (undefined)

AC, allocation concealment; ITT, use of intention-to-treat analysis (yes/no); MES, Melancholia Scale.

Lithium and lithium augmentation

Two trials considered the efficacy of lithium, one as monotherapy (Coppen *et al*, 1981) and the other as an augmentation of treatment with the tricyclic antidepressant nortriptyline (Sackeim *et al*, 2001).

Coppen *et al* (1981) randomised 38 patients currently receiving ECT to either lithium therapy or placebo. Patients began drug therapy while receiving ECT and before remission was established. Therefore the trial may have included people who were non-responders to ECT. Similarly, the number of drop-outs from the trial is not entirely clear (indeed, if there were any). Patients receiving lithium had significantly lower scores on the HRSD (16 items) than those receiving placebo at 52 weeks following initial recovery.

Sackeim *et al* (2001) randomised 28 patients to receive nortriptyline and lithium, 27 nortriptyline and 29 placebo for up to 24 weeks. As noted above, the main outcome measures were proportion of group relapsed and time to relapse. The relapse rate for patients who received nortriptyline plus lithium was 39% (95% CI 19 to 59) compared with 60% (95% CI 41 to 79) for those treated with nortriptyline alone. Using survival analysis, patients treated with nortriptyline plus lithium remained well significantly longer than those treated with placebo. Although those receiving nortriptyline became unwell more often during the trial, it is not clear whether augmentation with lithium was significantly more effective than nortriptyline alone.

Other strategies

Three other trials were identified: Grunhaus *et al* (2001) compared fluoxetine with fluoxetine plus melatonin, Kay *et al* (1970) considered amitriptyline versus diazepam and Meyers *et al* (2001) considered antipsychotic augmentation of antidepressant therapy.

Kay *et al* (1970) randomised patients to receive either amitriptyline (*n* = 59) or diazepam (*n* = 73) for 7 months following ECT treatment. The primary outcome measure was 'treatment failure', which was defined as a lack of satisfactory progress, relapse or failure for any other reason (e.g. overdose, serious side-effects). Subject groups were also compared on a number of rating scales. At the end of the trial a significant advantage was shown for amitriptyline-treated patents over those treated with diazepam in terms of treatment failure and in rating scale measurements (HRSD, Beck, Lubin).

Grunhaus *et al* (2001) randomised patients who had successfully responded to ECT to receive either fluoxetine and placebo (*n* = 15) or fluoxetine and melatonin (*n* = 20). At the end of the 3-month trial no differences were found in terms of relapse or in terms of mean rating scale measurements (various measures).

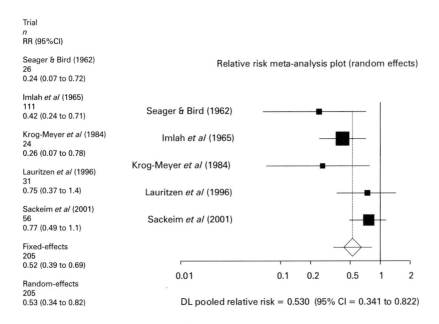

Trial
n
RR (95%CI)

Seager & Bird (1962)
26
0.24 (0.07 to 0.72)

Imlah *et al* (1965)
111
0.42 (0.24 to 0.71)

Krog-Meyer *et al* (1984)
24
0.26 (0.07 to 0.78)

Lauritzen *et al* (1996)
31
0.75 (0.37 to 1.4)

Sackeim *et al* (2001)
56
0.77 (0.49 to 1.1)

Fixed-effects
205
0.52 (0.39 to 0.69)

Random-effects
205
0.53 (0.34 to 0.82)

Relative risk meta-analysis plot (random effects)

DL pooled relative risk = 0.530 (95% CI = 0.341 to 0.822)

Figure 11.1 Meta-analysis of any antidepressant versus placebo (relative risk of relapse); DL, DerSimonian–Laird estimation of heterogeneity.

Meyers *et al* (2001) randomised patients who had successfully responded to ECT to either nortriptyline plus perphenazine (*n*=15) or nortriptyline plus placebo (*n*=13). No significant difference was found in terms of the proportion who relapsed (defined as meeting DSM–IV criteria for a major depressive episode or the development of delusional ideation). Patients in the antipsychotic plus nortriptyline groups experienced more extrapyramidal side-effects and falls than those treated with nortriptyline plus placebo.

Meta-analysis

Five RCTs evaluated the effects of an antidepressant treatment versus placebo on relapse. This comparison was considered using meta-analysis (Figure 11.1). Of the five trials, one used an SSRI and another considered both imipramine and phenelzine. In the latter trial, data from both the imipramine and phenelzine arms was combined before statistical combination. As four of five RCTs concerned tricyclic antidepressants, the comparison of tricyclic antidepressants with placebo is presented separately (Figure 11.2). Both analyses show statistically and clinically significant benefits of antidepressants. However, a plot of effect size against precision (Funnel plot; Fig. 11.3) appeared asymmetrical, which suggests the presence of publication bias.

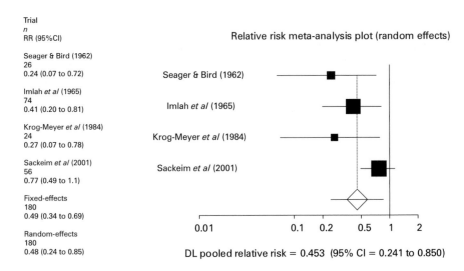

Trial
n
RR (95%CI)

Seager & Bird (1962)
26
0.24 (0.07 to 0.72)

Imlah *et al* (1965)
74
0.41 (0.20 to 0.81)

Krog-Meyer *et al* (1984)
24
0.27 (0.07 to 0.78)

Sackeim *et al* (2001)
56
0.77 (0.49 to 1.1)

Fixed-effects
180
0.49 (0.34 to 0.69)

Random-effects
180
0.48 (0.24 to 0.85)

Relative risk meta-analysis plot (random effects)

DL pooled relative risk = 0.453 (95% CI = 0.241 to 0.850)

Figure 11.2 Meta-analysis of tricyclic antidepressant versus placebo (relative risk of relapse); DL, DerSimonian–Laird estimation of heterogeneity.

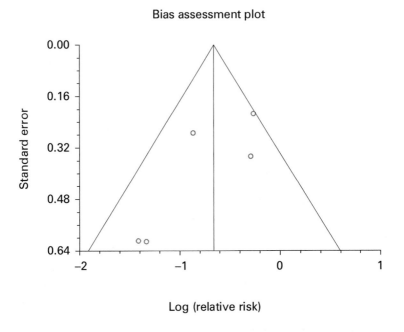

Bias assessment plot

Figure 11.3 Funnel plot for all randomised controlled trials of antidepressants versus placebo.

Discussion

The systematic review identified nine trials of the use of pharmaco-therapy to reduce relapse following ECT. The strongest evidence for therapeutic efficacy was found for antidepressants versus placebo, lithium augmentation of nortriptyline and for lithium as monotherapy. A single trial comparing amitriptyline with diazepam favoured amitrip-tyline and a further single trial of melatonin augmentation of fluoxetine found this strategy to be ineffective. Few of the included studies considered adverse effects.

The quality of trial reporting was generally poor and studies included as RCTs may not have been adequately conducted. This may have led to the effect of active treatment being overestimated. Further, the methodologies and outcomes used were heterogeneous. In particular, most studies randomised participants to receive pharmacological therapy before the completion of ECT and, indeed, before a therapeutic response had been established. In doing so, many trials may have randomised individuals who were not eligible to participate. In other cases these patients, and other drop-outs, were excluded and results are presented for completers only. Similarly, the lack of intention-to-treat analysis may have led to therapeutic effects being overestimated.

This meta-analysis of trials comparing antidepressants to placebo found a 47% reduction in relative risk with antidepressants. This is a substantial clinical effect and similar to the effect of continuation antidepressant therapy for depression (Loonen *et al*, 1991). Trial limitations may, however, have lead to bias and an overestimation of the treatment effect; this is possibly supported by the fact that the largest and best reported trial (Sackeim *et al*, 2001) found the smallest treatment effect. There was also evidence of funnel plot asymmetry, which suggests publication bias (i.e. that studies with findings of small, negative effects may not have been published).

Although little randomised evidence exists to guide the choice of drug, this review supports the current clinical practice of the prescription of maintenance pharmacotherapy following ECT. Furthermore, clinical practice in the 1960s and 1970s favoured ECT as a first-line therapy in depression (Sargant & Slater, 1964), in contrast to more recent times, when it has generally been reserved for more severe and treatment-resistant cases (American Psychiatric Association, 2001). Patients may therefore have a higher baseline risk of relapse following ECT now than they once did. Further trials of pharmacological, and perhaps non-pharmacological, interventions are therefore warranted. In the meantime, however, psychiatrists can prescribe and patients can take antidepressants (and/or lithium) after ECT in the knowledge that they are probably beneficial.

References

American Psychiatric Association (2001) *The Practice of Electroconvulsive Therapy: Recommendations for Treatment, Training and Privileging*. Washington, DC: APA.

Coppen, A., Abou-Saleh, M. T., Milln, P., *et al* (1981) Lithium continuation therapy following electroconvulsive therapy. *British Journal of Psychiatry*, **139**, 284–287.

Grunhaus, L., Hirschman, S., Dolberg, O. T., *et al* (2001) Coadministration of melatonin and fluoxetine does not improve the 3-month outcome following ECT. *Journal of ECT*, **17**, 124–128.

Imlah, N. W., Ryan, E. & Harrington, J. A. (1965) The influence of antidepressant drugs on the response to electroconvulsive therapy and on subsequent relapse rates. *Neuropsychopharmacology*, **4**, 438–442.

Kay, D. W., Fahy, T. & Garside, R. F. (1970) A seven-month double-blind trial of amitriptyline and diazepam in ECT-treated depressed patients. *British Journal of Psychiatry*, **117**, 667–671.

Krog-Meyer, I., Kirkegaard, C., Kijne, B., *et al* (1984) Prediction of relapse with the TRH test and prophylactic amitriptyline in 39 patients with endogenous depression. *American Journal of Psychiatry*, **141**, 945–948.

Lauritzen, L., Odgaard, K., Clemmesen, L., *et al* (1996) Relapse prevention by means of paroxetine in ECT-treated patients with major depression: a comparison with imipramine and placebo in medium-term continuation therapy. *Acta Psychiatrica Scandinavica*, **94**, 241–251.

Loonen, A. J., Peer, P. G. & Zwanikken, G. J. (1991) Continuation and maintenance therapy with antidepressive agents: meta-analysis of research. *Pharmacology Week Science*, **13**, 167–175.

Meyers, B. S., Klimstra, S. A., Gabriele, M., *et al* (2001) Continuation treatment of delusional depression in older adults. *American Journal of Geriatric Psychiatry*, **9**, 415–422.

O'Leary, D. A. & Lee, A. S. (1996) Seven-year prognosis in depression: mortality and readmission risk in the Nottingham ECT cohort. *British Journal of Psychiatry*, **169**, 423–429.

Sackeim, H. A., Haskett, R. F., Mulsant, B. H., *et al* (2001) Continuation pharmacotherapy in the prevention of relapse following electroconvulsive therapy: a randomized controlled trial. *Journal of the American Medical Association*, **285**, 1299–1307.

Sargant, W. & Slater, E. (1964) *An Introduction to Physical Methods of Treament in Psychiatry*. Baltimore: Williams & Wilkins.

Seager, C. P. & Bird, R. L. (1962) Imipramine with electrical treatment in depression – a controlled trial. *Journal of Mental Science*, **108**, 704–707.

CHAPTER 12

Psychotropic drug treatment during and after ECT

Allan I. F. Scott

The previous edition of the present book included a review of the prescription of psychotropic drugs with ECT; it noted that clinical studies of the topic were few and that most research had been done in animals, usually rats (Curran & Freeman, 1995). The included clinical studies were largely case reports. One of the tenets of evidence-based medicine is that, like therapeutic effects, the risks of adverse effects are best estimated from a randomised controlled trial (RCT). This was one important reason that the two systematic reviews presented in Chapters 10 and 11 were commissioned, and it was disappointing to observe how little evidence was available from RCTs. The present chapter reviews the previous recommendations in light of the findings from the systematic reviews and other relevant research. Many of the recommendations remain valid and relevant.

Psychotropic drugs and ECT technique

Most patients treated with ECT take psychotropic drugs and many of these may have significant effects on both the seizure threshold and the seizure duration. Several recommendations were made about interactions that might require modification to ECT technique; for example, a low electrical 'dose' would be indicated in patients pre-medicated with a selective serotonin reuptake inhibitor (SSRI) or the lithium ion, but higher doses might be required in patients taking drugs with anti-convulsant properties. An implicit assumption was made that most clinics use a fixed electrical dose rather than adjust the dose for the individual patient. Even today, only a minority of ECT clinics make any attempt to quantify the seizure threshold at the start of the course of treatment (see Chapter 16). It may be that the risks of either prolonged cerebral seizure activity or compromised therapeutic efficacy would be reduced or avoided by the adoption of an ECT technique where the seizure threshold is empirically measured at the first treatment, though this does not seem to have been tested.

Benzodiazepine drugs

There remains a valid concern based both on laboratory and clinical evidence that the concomitant intake of a benzodiazepine drug may compromise the therapeutic efficacy of ECT, because this group of drugs has powerful anticonvulsant properties. There has been only one RCT of relevance, and this was conducted more than 30 years ago (Kay *et al*, 1970); it was not designed to investigate the seizure-inhibiting properties of the concomitant intake of a benzodiazepine drug, but the findings suggested that diazepam may reduce the antidepressant efficacy of ECT (see Chapter 10).

Recommendations

- Wherever clinically possible, the concomitant prescription of benzodiazepine drugs should be avoided during a course of ECT.
- If a hypnotic drug is clinically indicated at night, then it would be good practice to consider the use of a non-benzodiazepine drug.
- Long-established benzodiazepine drug use should not be stopped suddenly just a few days before a course of ECT because there is the risk of a dramatic lowering of seizure threshold. If the dose cannot be gradually reduced and stopped before the administration of ECT, it may be better to continue the drug during ECT, perhaps in reduced dosage.

Antidepressant drugs

The limited evidence from RCTs suggests that the antidepressant effect of ECT may be marginally augmented by the co-prescription of an antidepressant drug, and without major risks (see Chapter 10). Two major caveats are required, one about efficacy and one about safety. First, evidence from RCTs shows that the prescription of an antidepressant drug after a successful course of ECT substantially reduces the risk of early relapse (see Chapter 11). It may be that the prescription of an antidepressant drug before the end of a course of ECT simply augments this prophylactic effect rather than the antidepressant effect of ECT itself. Second, there continue to be case reports of prolonged cerebral seizure activity putatively linked to either the co-prescription of an antidepressant drug or the abrupt discontinuation of an antidepressant drug, usually an SSRI. It may therefore be prudent to repeat the previous recommendation that a low electrical dose be used during the first administration of ECT to patients who have been premedicated with SSRIs.

Recommendations

- An antidepressant drug should not be abruptly discontinued before ECT, particularly one with a short half-life or one of the SSRIs.
- Monoamine oxidase inhibitors do not need to be discontinued before ECT, but the anaesthetist should be informed in advance that the patient is taking one.
- It is probably better to prescribe an effective antidepressant drug at least before the end of a course of treatment, if only to provide adequate early prophylaxis.
- In elderly patients, or patients with pre-existing cardiac disease, potential cardiotoxicity should influence the choice of drug.
- In patients premedicated with an SSRI, it would be prudent to start with a low electrical dose (25–50 mC) at the first treatment.

Lithium

There have been conflicting opinions about both the efficacy and safety of the lithium ion prescribed during a course of ECT. The likeliest explanation for the lack of consensus is that most of the relevant literature consists only of case reports. There has been only one RCT of the co-prescription of lithium carbonate, which was completed more than 20 years ago (Coppen *et al*, 1981). A tentative interpretation of the findings would be that the early introduction of the lithium ion may reduce the risk of early relapse (see Chapters 10 and 11).

Much of the conflict concerns whether or not the body of case reports associate the co-administration of the lithium ion and adverse effects such as prolonged cerebral seizure activity or prolonged dis-orientation (see review by Mukherjee, 1993). It remains prudent, but sufficient, to suggest that, like premedication with an SSRI, only a low electrical dose be used at the first treatment because the co-administration of lithium reduces the seizure threshold.

In the management of bipolar disorder, the discontinuation of lithium before ECT may generate risks. While the intake of the lithium ion reduces the risk of future episodes of illness, its abrupt discontinuation increases the risk of precipitating new episodes of elation; it has been recommended that lithium prophylaxis be taken for at least 2 years to ensure that the benefit of prophylaxis outweighs the risk of relapse associated with its discontinuation (Goodwin, 2003).

Recommendations

- The co-administration of the lithium ion is not a contraindication to ECT.

- Preliminary evidence suggests that the early introduction of the lithium ion reduces the likelihood of early relapse of depressive illness after ECT.
- The co-administration of the lithium ion with ECT may be one risk factor among several for adverse effects such as prolonged cerebral seizure activity. It may be prudent to start with a low electrical dose (25–50 mC) at the first treatment.

Anti-epileptic drugs

These might be prescribed during a course of ECT either for the treatment of epilepsy itself or for their putative mood-stabilising effects. In either case there is little clinical evidence to guide practice. If an anti-epileptic drug is prescribed to treat epilepsy, then its prescription should continue throughout the course of ECT. This is not a controversial suggestion, but there is still no consensus about the co-prescription of anti-epileptic drugs for mood stabilisation. The previous edition of this handbook suggested that they continue to be prescribed, presumably because this helps reduce the risk of early relapse after ECT. Other practitioners view this group of drugs like the benzodiazepine drugs, and try at least to reduce the daily dose before ECT. Still others leave the dose unchanged before ECT, at least initially, although they are prepared to titrate the daily dose downwards if seizure induction becomes problematic during the course of ECT.

Recommendations

- If used to treat epilepsy, the prescription of an anti-epileptic drug should continue throughout the course of ECT.
- If used as a mood stabiliser, no evidence-based recommendation can be made; on balance, it may be better to continue the prescription during the course of ECT.
- Anti-epileptic drugs may raise the seizure threshold, shorten seizure duration and modify the convulsion; ECT titration schedules will therefore have to take account of the co-administration of anti-epileptic drugs.
- If the induction of seizures becomes problematic during the course of ECT, the prescribed daily dose may need to be reduced.

Antipsychotic drugs

The evidence from RCTs was reviewed in Chapter 4 for schizophrenia and in Chapter 10 for depressive illness. The recommendation for schizophrenia was that ECT is regarded as an option only when antipsychotic drug treatment has failed to bring about sufficient improvement. It has not been shown that there is a synergistic effect between ECT and antipsychotic drugs in such treatment-resistant cases. In depressive illness, the limited evidence did not suggest any synergistic effect. The previous recommendations require additional comment only for the use of clozapine.

Epileptic seizures are a recognised adverse effect of clozapine. There have been case reports of either prolonged or tardive seizures associated with the simultaneous or recent administration of clozapine with ECT (see Bloch *et al*, 1996). There are now substantially more case reports which suggest that clozapine can be administered safety with ECT (see Chapter 4).

The manufacturer of clozapine in the UK suggests that the drug be withheld for 12 hours before any general anaesthetic; the next dose after surgery can be given at the usual time and at the usual dose if the patient's vital signs are stable.

Recommendations

- A small dose of a sedative antipsychotic drug may be preferred to a benzodiazepine drug if a hypnotic drug is indicated.
- The manufacturer of clozapine suggests that the drug is withheld for 12 hours before any general anaesthetic.
- Clozapine may lower the seizure threshold, and it may be prudent to start with a low electrical dose (25–50 mC) at the first treatment.

Caffeine

It has been suggested that the co-administration of caffeine, an adenosine antagonist, might augment the therapeutic effects of ECT by prolonging cerebral seizure activity. Interest in this suggestion soon disappeared, however, when an RCT found that the intravenous injection of caffeine 5 minutes before ECT prolonged cerebral seizure activity by about one-third, but had no effect at all on the seizure threshold (McCall *et al*, 1993). It was argued that the length of the seizure was not related to outcome and there would be no therapeutic benefit if caffeine did not lower the seizure threshold (see Chapter 15 for discussion of seizure threshold).

Recommendation

- The co-administration of caffeine is unlikely to augment the therapeutic effects of ECT.

Continuation treatment after ECT

It has been established for more than 30 years that there is a high risk of relapse in the first few weeks after successful ECT if patients are left untreated. It is already a recommendation that the minimum requirement after successful ECT is for continuation medical treatment at a full therapeutic dose for at least 6 months. In depressive illness, the prevention of early relapse is becoming a greater challenge for the reasons discussed in Chapter 2. Continuation treatment was not routine clinical practice around the time of the previous edition of this handbook (Riddle & Scott, 1995). The challenge of managing the severe and treatment-resistant illnesses for which ECT is now reserved would suggest that vigorous medical treatment has become routine, but there are accounts from the USA that this is not so (McCall *et al*, 2002); in particular, Sackeim *et al* (2000) reported that about 20% of depressed patients did not receive a therapeutic course of antidepressant drug treatment in the 12 months after a course of ECT. It is not known if this is a problem of prescription or adherence, but it clearly merits further study.

Six months of continuation treatment must be seen as the bare minimum. At least 12 months of continuation treatment has been recommended for late-life depressive illness (Baldwin *et al*, 2003). Most contemporary patients treated with ECT suffer from recurrent illness and are likely to be candidates both for more intensive continuation treatment and for longer-term prophylactic treatment, to reduce the risk of future episodes of illness. Evidence-based recommendations for prophylactic treatment are available for depressive illness (Anderson *et al*, 2000), bipolar disorder (Goodwin, 2003) and schizophrenia (American Psychiatric Association, 1997).

Gaps in the evidence

Unfortunately, there is a lack of relevant clinical research about important aspects of continuation treatment after ECT for depressive illness, the commonest contemporary indication. There is no agreement about how to manage patients who were prescribed ECT because they had not improved sufficiently with antidepressant drug treatment. There is one school of thought that treatment with ECT, even if it does not bring about complete remission of symptoms, brings about neurochemical changes that make a depressive illness more likely to respond to antidepressant drugs, including those that have previously been ineffective (Shapira *et al*, 1988). Other commentators disagree and recommend that after a successful course of ECT a switch is made to a different class of antidepressant drug rather than continue or reintroduce a drug from a class that has already provided ineffective in the index episode (American Psychiatric Association, 2001).

There is inadequate research to state clearly that one class of antidepressant drug is more efficacious than another in continuation treatment (see Chapter 11). There is, though, evidence that tricyclic antidepressant drugs such as amitriptyline are more efficacious than SSRIs in patients who require admission to hospital (Anderson *et al*, 2000). It is an extrapolation of untested validity, but it may be prudent to consider such drugs as the treatment of choice in patients at high risk of relapse of depression. There is also preliminary evidence that the addition of lithium carbonate to continuation antidepressant drug treatment further reduces the risk of relapse (see Chapter 11).

There is no directly applicable evidence to guide the management of delusional depressive illness after ECT. Such patients may be candidates for an augmentation strategy, in this case with an antipsychotic drug. Once remission has been established for 4 months, it may be reasonable gradually to reduce the dose of antipsychotic drug (Rothschild & Duval, 2003).

There has not been an RCT of the management of depressed patients who have responded only partially, if at all, to ECT. It may be reasonable that treatment follows the same principles as for those patients thought to be at high risk of early relapse, that is, treatment with a tricyclic drug such as amitriptyline plus a relevant augmentation strategy. There has similarly been no clinical trial to assess the efficacy or effectiveness of a psychological or psychosocial treatment, either as monotherapy or as an augmentation strategy.

Where vigorous continuation treatment has previously proved ineffective or intolerable, ECT itself may be considered as continuation treatment (see Chapter 9). This option has been inadequately researched and is controversial (see Chapter 1). The American Psychiatric Association (2001) has already called for the investigation of novel strategies to try to meet the clinical challenge of caring for patients at high risk of relapse after ECT.

Recommendations

- Continuation treatment with doses of medicine known to be therapeutic are essential for at least 6 months after successful ECT.
- Many contemporary patients will be at high risk of relapse and therefore candidates for vigorous continuation treatment, often involving augmentation strategies.
- It may be good practice to use this approach also for patients who have not yet fully recovered with ECT.
- Many patients who have suffered from recurrent episodes of illness will be candidates for longer-term prophylactic or maintenance treatment to reduce the likelihood of new episodes of illness.

References

American Psychiatric Association (1997) Practice guideline for the treatment of patients with schizophrenia. *American Journal of Psychiatry*, **154** (suppl. 4).

American Psychiatric Association (2001) *The Practice of Electroconvulsive Therapy: Recommendations for Treatment, Training and Priviledging* (2nd edn). Washington, DC: American Psychiatric Press.

Anderson, I. M., Nutt, D. J. & Deakin, J. F. (2000) Evidence-based guidelines for treating depressive disorders with antidepressants: a revision of the 1993 British Association for Psychopharmacology guidelines. *Journal of Psychopharmacology*, **14**, 3–20.

Baldwin, R. C., Anderson, D., Black, S., *et al* (2003) Guidline for the management of late-life depression in primary care. *International Journal of Geriatric Psychiatry*, **18**, 829–838.

Bloch, Y., Pollack, N. & Mor, I. (1996) Should the administration of ECT during clozapine therapy be contraindicated? *British Journal of Psychiatry*, **169**, 253–254.

Coppen, A., Abou-Saleh, M. T., Milln, P., *et al* (1981) Lithium continuation therapy following electroconvulsive therapy. *British Journal of Psychiatry*, **139**, 284–287.

Curran, S. & Freeman, C. P. (1995) ECT and drugs. In *The ECT Handbook* (ed. C. P. Freeman). London: Royal College of Psychiatrists.

Goodwin, G. M., for the Consensus Group of the British Association for Psychopharmacology (2003) Evidence-based guidelines for treating bipolar disorder. *Journal of Psychopharmacology*, **17**, 149–173.

Kay, D. W., Fahy, T. & Garside, R. F. (1970) A seven-month double-blind trial of amitriptyline and diazepam in ECT-treated depressed patients. *British Journal of Psychiatry*, **117**, 667–671.

McCall, W. V., Reid, S., Rosenquist, P., *et al* (1993) A reappraisal of the role of caffeine in ECT. *American Journal of Psychiatry*, **150**, 1543–1545.

McCall, W. V., Dunn, A., Rosen, P. B., *et al* (2002) Markedly suprathreshold right unilateral ECT versus minimally suprathreshold bilateral ECT: antidepressant and memory effects. *Journal of ECT*, **18**, 126–129.

Mukherjee, S. (1993) Combined ECT and lithium therapy. *Convulsive Therapy*, **9**, 274–284.

Riddle, W. J. R. & Scott, A. I. F. (1995) Relapse after successful electroconvulsive therapy: the use and impact of continuation antidepressant drug treatment. *Human Psychopharmacology*, **10**, 201–206.

Rothschild, A. J. & Duval, S. E. (2003) How long should patients with psychotic depression stay on their antipsychotic medication? *Journal of Clinical Psychiatry*, **64**, 390–396.

Sackeim, H. A., Prudic, J., Devanand, D. P., *et al* (2000) A prospective, randomized, double-blind comparison of bilateral and right unilateral ECT at different stimulus intensities. *Archives of General Psychiatry*, **57**, 425–434.

Shapira, B., Kindler, S. & Lerer, B. (1988) Medication outcome in ECT-resistant depression. *Convulsive Therapy*, **4**, 192–198.

Part III
The administration of ECT

CHAPTER 13

The ECT suite

Chris P. Freeman and Grace M. Fergusson

Ideally, there should be a designated area for ECT within each general psychiatry unit; this is recommended on the basis of patient convenience and economy of nurse staffing. However, it is recognised that, with the numbers of patients undergoing ECT falling, there is an increasing trend for psychiatric services to share one facility in an attempt to maintain standards of anaesthetic and psychiatric practice within the confines of a National Health Service budget.

Suite layout

The design of the ECT suite will depend on the type of service provided. The minimum requirement for a local unit with small patient numbers is two rooms: a treatment room and a recovery room. An ECT unit where patients would be required to wait before treatment will need a waiting room in addition. A suite providing ECT to neighbouring psychiatric units should ideally include an ECT office and a final post-ECT waiting area.

The waiting room should be comfortable and informal. Patients' arrival should be booked to provide a smooth throughput with the minimum amount of waiting time. The room should provide a relaxing environment with distractions, and toilet facilities should be available.

Accessible from the waiting area should be a treatment room, where the patient is assisted onto a trolley or bed and prepared for treatment. This room should be well lit and contain all the equipment necessary for routine and emergency treatment. It should be big enough to allow unrestricted staff movements. Adequate work surfaces and hot and cold water should be available.

There should be good sound-proofing between the waiting area and treatment room, and waiting patients should not be able to see into the treatment room each time the door is opened.

The recovery area must be large enough to accommodate easily the trolleys and associated monitors of all the patients who are regaining consciousness, and there should be enough room for recovery nursing staff to work in. The size will therefore vary according to the activity levels of the ECT suite and should be calculated on the basis of the maximum number of unconscious patients expected at any one session, bearing in mind that the average time for recovery varies from 5 to 30 minutes.

There should be a direct link between the treatment and recovery areas, through a doorway wide enough to admit a trolley or bed easily; this will allow ready access for the anaesthetic team and emergency equipment if necessary. Telephone access should be provided in case of the need to summon help. Patients remain in this primary recovery area until they are able to walk and are reoriented.

From the recovery area the patients may be escorted to the post-ECT waiting area, to await transport and where refreshments can be provided. This room should be designed to accommodate all patients and escorting nurses in a relaxed environment.

A separate office is required for the administration of a busy ECT clinic or one serving neighbouring psychiatric units.

Regionalisation of ECT services

A recent Department of Health review in England and Wales and the National Audit of ECT in Scotland (Freeman et al, 2000; Department of Health, 2003; Fergusson et al, 2004) have both confirmed a significant fall over the past 10 years in the numbers of patients who receive ECT. This, together with an anaesthetic requirement for increased staffing and monitoring, has resulted in a move towards regional centres serving several catchment populations. There are certain advantages and disadvantages inherent in this development.

Advantages

- Expensive anaesthetic monitoring and ECT equipment are shared.
- Similary shared are suitably trained personnel – anaesthetist, operating department personnel (ODP), psychiatrist.
- Regional centres will give sufficient numbers of treatments for staff to maintain their skills.
- They provide adequate training opportunities for all sectors of staff.

Disadvantages

- They may be inconvenient to reach for some patients.
- Trained nurse escorts are required in satellite units when patients are transferred for ECT.
- Problems of clearly assigning clinical reponsibility and ensuring the safe transport of patients to and from the ECT clinic.

- There is a need to consider the transfer of care for very frail or physically sick patients.

Staffing

Nursing staff

The number of nursing staff required at any one ECT session will depend on the number of patients undergoing treatment and the type of service provided. In any case, the following conditions apply:

- There must be one trained nurse, with managerial responsibility, in overall charge of the ECT session.
- One trained nurse should be in charge at each stage of the treatment process.
- There should be one trained nurse, known to the patient, accompanying them throughout.
- There should be one nurse, trained in cardiopulmonary resuscitation, with each unconscious patient.
- Additional nurses should be available to help in the recovery areas of a busy clinic or if required for backup.

See also Appendix VII.

Medical staff

The following are required:

- a senior psychiatrist
- a senior anaesthetist (see Chapter 14)
- ODP or equivalent whose sole role is to assist the anaesthetist.

Equipment for the ECT suite

The following are required:

- *An ECT machine.* A brief-pulse, constant-current ECT machine is required with a wide output range and a facility for electro-encephalography. It is important that there is a back-up arrangement in case the ECT machine develops a fault. This might be with a medical physics department or a neighbouring ECT service, to provide an ECT machine before the next treatment day. Appropriate electrodes and conducting gel or solution will also be required.
- *Trolley or bed with firm base.* This should have a tilt facility and cot sides. One per patient until recovery is required.
- *Oxygen.* This should be delivered by intermittent positive pressure ventilation from either a cylinder with a reserve or an anaesthetic

machine, with appropriate circuits for supply and scavenging. There should be one face mask per patient.

- *Suction*. Suction machine plus backup, tubing and catheters must be available.
- *Sundries*. These will include disposable gloves, mouth gags, airways, syringes, needles, intravenous cannulae, tape, scissors, swabs, skin cleanser/degreaser and weighing scales.
- *Disposal*. Appropriate disposal facilities are required for sharps and clinical waste.
- *Monitoring*. For the purposes of monitoring the patient during the administration of ECT, the following will be required:
  - log-book of patients receiving ECT
  - blood glucose testing kit
  - stopwatch or clock with minute hand plus electroencephalograph for determining seizure length
  - manual or automatic sphygmomanometer for measuring blood pressure
  - electrocardiographic monitor with electrodes
  - pulse oximeter to determine oxygen saturation
  - capnograph to measure end-tidal carbon dioxide levels in an intubated patient.
- *Anaesthetic drugs*. These will be as agreed by local protocol in consultation with the anaesthetist. (Chapter 14 considers the anaesthetic equipment and procedures in more detail.)
- *Emergency drugs and equipment*. These are detailed under a separate section below.

Recovery room

In the recovery room the following are required:

- a pulse oximeter for monitoring each unconscious patient
- a blood pressure monitor, as above
- an oxygen source, as above
- suction equipment, as above
- emergency drugs and equipment (see below).

Chapter 14 gives further information on the recovery room, inrelation to anaesthesia.

Emergency drugs and equipment

Emergency drugs and equipment should be available in the treatment room and easily accessible to all other ECT areas during treatment sessions. These will include:

- a cardiac defibrillator
- a laryngoscope, plus a backup, as well as laryngeal masks, endotracheal tubes and associated connectors
- intravenous infusion sets, fluids, stand and associated sundries
- a stethoscope
- a thermometer
- ice packs
- an emergency drug box, the contents of which will have been agreed by local protocol.

Maintenance

An agreement should be in place for the regular maintenance of all equipment, either with the machine manufacturer or with the medical physics department.

References

Department of Health (2003) Electroconvulsive therapy: survey covering the period from January 2002 to March 2002, England. London: Department of Health.

Fergusson, G. M., Cullen, L. A., Freeman, C. P. L. *et al* (2004) Electroconvulsive therapy in Scottish clinical practice: a national audit of demographics, standards and outcome. *Journal of ECT*, **20**, 166–173.

Freeman, C. P. L., Hendry, J. & Fergusson, G. (2000) *National Audit of Electroconvulsive Therapy in Scotland. Final Report.* Available at www.sean.org.uk/report/report00.php.

Anaesthesia for ECT

C. John Bowley and Heather A. C. Walker

Anaesthesia for ECT must be given by an *experienced* anaesthetist, capable of managing potential complications at a site possibly remote from the main hospital, aided by a suitably trained assistant (Association of Anaesthetists of Great Britain and Ireland, 1998). Regular consultant input is essential. Each department involved in ECT should allocate responsibility for providing the associated anaesthetic service to a consultant anaesthetist who can liaise with the psychiatrists (Simpson & Lynch, 1998). This individual can supervise the assessment of patients, offer advice on their preparation for general anaesthesia and arrange the provision of the necessary anaesthetic and monitoring equipment, as well as adequate numbers of trained anaesthetic assistants, recovery staff and appropriately experienced anaesthetists.

Pre-ECT assessment

Initial assessment may be performed by the psychiatrist or an ECT clinic senior nurse or nurse practitioner. Guidelines, in the form of a checklist, may help staff to identify potential problems with anaesthesia. Medical history should highlight whether the patient has a condition which may affect anaesthesia. Of particular relevance are (Rice *et al*, 1994):

- angina
- recent myocardial infarction
- cerebrovascular accident (CVA)
- diabetes
- hypertension
- hiatus hernia
- known drug allergies
- adverse reactions to previous anaesthetics.

Physical examination should expose any evidence of cardiac failure, severe valvular disease or unstable dysrhythmia, uncontrolled hypertension, significant infection, poor dentition, obesity, marked cachexia or factors that might prejudice airway management, such as arthritis, particularly of the neck or jaw.

The patient's blood pressure (BP), weight and urinalysis should be recorded.

Investigations

Any of the following may be performed, but only as clinically indicated:

- full blood count – on most patients
- sickle test – on Afro-Caribbean, Eastern Mediterranean, Asian and Middle Eastern patients
- urea and electrolytes (U&E) – for patients taking lithium (for whom determination of lithium levels may be advisable), diuretics or other vasoactive/cardiac drugs, those with diabetes and those with renal disease
- liver function tests – on patients with cachexia, a history of alcoholism, drug abuse or recent overdose
- international normalised ratio (INR) – for patients taking anti-coagulants
- hepatitis B antigen status – on known drug abusers
- blood sugar levels – if urinalysis is positive
- electrocardiogram – on patients with known cardiovascular, respiratory or renal disease, irregular pulse or heart murmur, hypertension, those with diabetes aged over 40, and all patients over 50
- chest X-ray – for patients with suspected chest infection, cardiomegaly, congestive cardiac failure, pulmonary embolism (PE) or who have had recent falls (because of the possibility of fractured ribs)
- lung function tests – for patients with severe chronic obstructive airways diseases, or shortness of breath at rest
- a pregnancy test – if appropriate.

A list of the standard investigations required before a new course of ECT is begun should be agreed with the local anaesthetic department.

All results must be available in the notes for anaesthetic review before ECT.

Fitness for ECT/general anaesthesia

Patients whose condition or results give cause for concern should be referred for specific anaesthetic assessment, well in advance of the proposed ECT, to avoid last-minute cancellations. In practice more patients are cancelled for failure to fast (see below) than through ill health.

The relatively few contraindications to ECT include the following:

- uncontrolled cardiac failure
- deep venous thrombosis – until anticoagulated (to reduce risk of PE)
- acute respiratory infection
- recent myocardial infarction (within 3 months and depending on severity)
- recent CVA (within 1 month and depending on severity)
- raised intracranial pressure/untreated cerebral aneurysm
- unstable major fracture
- untreated phaeochromocytoma.

In all cases a balance must be struck between the risks of anaesthesia/ECT, those of any concurrent medical conditions and the risks of untreated depression. Occasionally ECT may be life-saving, and under such circumstances there may be no absolute contraindications (Kelly & Zisselman, 2000).

Old age alone does not preclude ECT.

Patients with implanted pacemakers can receive ECT, with full electrocardiographic monitoring (Pinski & Trohman, 1995; Pornnoppadol & Isenberg, 1998). Implantable cardioverter defibrillators should have defibrillation and antitachycardia functions deactivated before ECT (Diprose & Pierce, 2001).

The administration of ECT is possible in pregnancy, depending upon gestation: early risks of miscarriage give way to those of supine hypotension and oesophageal reflux, which may require pre-treatment with H_2 antagonists, sodium citrate and/or endotracheal intubation. Treatment should be planned in consultation with the patient's obstetrician, when consideration should be given to methods of foetal monitoring and whether the presence of a midwife, especially in the latter stages of pregnancy, would be appropriate.

Patients who are thought to be at high risk (ASA III or above, i.e. patients with moderate systemic disease with definite functional limitation, affecting lifestyle, Saklad, 1941) should not be treated in remote locations; consideration should be given to transferring these patients to a more suitable environment, such as a theatre suite or its recovery area. Should initial treatment prove uneventful, then it may be possible to continue the course at the original (remote) location, after full consultation between the members of the ECT team.

Preparation of the patient for ECT

A checklist should be completed for all patients to verify:

- identity (patients should be provided with a name band, including hospital number)

- ward/out-patient
- legal status
- consent
- fasting state
- presence/removal of dentures, jewellery, hearing aids and contact lenses
- details of any premedication
- transport requirements
- date of last ECT and general anaesthesia.

Unless specifically stated, all regular medications, with the exception of insulin, should be taken, not less than 2 hours before treatment, with sips of water if necessary. Otherwise patients should take no food for 6 hours and drink only moderate volumes of clear fluids until 2 hours before treatment.

The patients should be given the opportunity to pass urine. Blood pressure, pulse, temperature and weight should be recorded. For known diabetics a blood glucose estimate should be performed immediately before each treatment.

Checklists must be signed and dated by the ECT suite staff.

Day-care patients, or their carers, must sign a declaration that the patient will not drive for at least 24 hours, will be accompanied home and have appropriate responsible adult supervision for the night after each treatment.

Any written advice on the post-treatment period should be given to both the patient and the escort.

Materials and equipment in the ECT suite reception area

The following should be available in the reception area (see also Chapter 13):

- blank checklists
- scales to weigh the patient
- automated non-invasive blood pressure (NIBP) monitoring or sphygmomanometer and stethoscope
- patient thermometer
- blood glucose testing kit
- containers for personal belongings and so on
- access to toilet facilities.

The main treatment area should be of adequate size, well lit and be equipped with tilting trolley(s) with cot sides that can be padded. This will be used for treatment and recovery until the patient can sit in a chair. An easy-slip device should be in position under the patient to facilitate turning. The room should have a clock with a second hand.

A secure drug storage cupboard, a small fridge and hand-washing facilities should be immediately available.

A full anaesthetic machine is usually not required but there must be a flow-controlled oxygen supply, either by pipeline or cylinder (plus reserve). A Bain or Waters circuit will be needed to support ventilation. Airway circuits should be checked for function and patency before use. Suction of sufficient power must be available with Yankauer ends and soft suction catheters.

A system of resupply of disposables such as gloves, syringes, needles, cannulae, tape, electrodes, airways and mouth guards should be established, together with approved containers for the safe disposal of contaminated material.

Reusable airway equipment should incorporate disposable filters.

Monitoring

Monitoring of NIBP, electrocardiogram, pulse oximetry and end-tidal carbon dioxide are mandatory (Association of Anaesthetists of Great Britain and Ireland, 2000).

A peripheral nerve stimulator may be useful.

Some ECT machines incorporate recording of the electroencephalogram (EEG), which can provide useful data about seizure duration.

Monitors with battery packs can be useful should patient transfer be necessary.

Written records of monitor readings should be kept.

Emergency/resuscitation equipment

The emergency/resuscitation equipment should include the following:

- A selection of airways, laryngoscopes (possibly McCoy), a range of endotracheal tubes and connectors, a bougie and laryngeal masks or other 'difficult airway' device(s) may be helpful. Many departments are equipped with single-use 'difficult airway' boxes with equipment for managing respiratory emergencies such as pneumothorax or upper-airway obstruction.
- A selection of intravenous (IV) fluids, giving sets, pressure infuser and drip stand should be available.
- Cardiac arrest and other emergency drugs are usually supplied in single-use containers with locally agreed contents.
- A defibrillator, which should be checked (and this recorded) before each session.

Resuscitation guidelines should be available in each ECT suite and periodic emergency-resuscitation 'drills' practised.

Concurrent medication

Concurrent therapy can be considered under two headings: general medication and specific psychiatric medication. Both have the potential to modify seizure thresholds. Anticonvulsants, hypnotics and membrane stabilisers tend to raise the seizure threshold, while preparations containing theophyllines can have the opposite effect.

Patients' concurrent medication is usually of a protective nature, such as anti-hypertensives, anti-anginals, anti-dysrhythmics, bronchodilators and/or antacid/anti-reflux therapy. These should be maintained and can usually be given safely, up to 2 hours before ECT, with sips of water if necessary. Those receiving long-term steroids may need supplementary doses and those on anticholinesterase therapy for glaucoma may require modification of the choice of muscle relaxant. Patients with diabetes who require insulin should attend early in the day and should have medication withheld until after recovery. H_2 receptor antagonists and antacids should be prescribed for those at risk of oesophageal reflux (Kadar *et al*, 2002). A strict fasting regimen of 6 hours for food and 2 hours for clear fluids must be observed.

Concurrent psychiatric medication can have a significant effect upon ECT. Benzodiazepines are anticonvulsant and should be avoided if possible, but there are risks associated with their sudden withdrawal. Some authorities have suggested short-term reversal with flumazenil if their presence is considered to be a limiting factor in the success of ECT, but experience is limited (Bailine *et al*, 1994; Hanania, 1995). Tricyclics tend to be proconvulsant, but there is little evidence of any detrimental effect on ECT. Selective serotonin reuptake inhibitors (SSRIs) tend to reduce seizure threshold and may be associated with prolonged seizures. Fluoxetine has a long half-life and it is recommended that ECT treatment be started at low dosage (25–50 mC). Monoamine oxidase inhibitors increase seizure threshold and it is essential that the anaesthetist is aware that the patient is taking this class of medication or has done so within the previous 2 weeks. Lithium reduces seizure threshold and serum levels should be checked regularly and kept within a moderate range (0.4–1 mmol/l). Selective inhibitors of the reuptake of serotonin and noradrenaline can reduce seizure threshold and cause hypertension. Neuroleptics tend to be proconvulsant at low dosage but increase seizure thresholds at higher dosage.

Conduct of anaesthesia

Anaesthesia for ECT not only enables the procedure but also has a major influence on its efficacy. Moreover, during a course of ECT patients frequently present for several anaesthetics within a short period of time, and can be emotionally labile and receiving treatment for other medical conditions.

The objective of anaesthesia is to provide the shortest period of unconsciousness necessary to cover muscle relaxation, the electrical stimulus and resultant seizure. A rapid return to full consciousness and orientation is desirable.

Premedication is usually unnecessary but remains at the discretion of the anaesthetist, who must be satisfied with the patient's fitness for the procedure and be aware of the patient's response to any previous sessions of ECT and the doses of anaesthetic agents used (Mayur *et al*, 1998).

The patient is reassured as necessary and asked to lie on the trolley. Then the electrocardiograph, pulse oximeter and NIBP monitor are attached; initial readings are recorded and intravenous access secured. Any short-acting agents needed to modify the anticipated hypertensive response to ECT may be administered at this point and, if necessary, pre-oxygenation is begun (Castelli *et al*, 1995).

Induction agents

The dose of induction agent is, at least initially, related to the patient's weight but subsequent doses should be modified in the light of the response to ECT and any changing or induced seizure threshold.

Propofol (0.75–2.5 mg/kg) is increasing in popularity. It is thought to reduce seizure duration but improve cardiovascular stability. Seizure duration in any case may be only marginally related to the clinical efficacy of ECT (Fear *et al*, 1994). Propofol confers little advantage in terms of long- and medium-term recovery, does not appear to cause any reduction in postictal cognitive deficit and its injection can be painful. The addition of a small amount of lidocaine or the use of propofol emulsion to reduce pain on injection does not seem to have any adverse effect on seizure activity. Propofol's use is likely to increase as more data become available.

Thiopental (2–5 mg/kg) has the disadvantage of having to be reconstituted into solution and haemodynamic parameters appear less well attenuated when compared with propofol (Kadoi *et al*, 2003). Its recovery characteristics do not appear to be particularly disadvantageous, but it has been suggested that postictal dysrhythmias may be more common with thiopental than with propofol.

Etomidate (0.15–0.3 mg/kg) is used in some centres and produces longer seizures than the more traditional agents. It has proved effective in patients in whom it has been found to be difficult to produce any seizure activity or who demonstrate brief or abortive seizures (Avramov *et al*, 1995). The haemodynamic responses tend to be greater in comparison with other commonly used induction agents.

Ketamine is largely unsuitable for routine use owing to its potential emergence phenomena, long recovery period and tendency to produce hypertension (Rasmussen *et al*, 1996). It has been used successfully, however, when it has otherwise proved particularly difficult to produce any seizure activity despite maximal charge delivery.

Induction is usually by intravenous injection, although, with the availability of sevoflurane, inhalation induction is now a real possibility, providing the appropriate equipment and scavenging are available. It may be an especially useful alternative for patients with poor venous access, although further experience is needed. Its use has been reported in the third trimester of pregnancy to attenuate uterine contraction following ECT.

Whichever induction agent is chosen, it is probably unwise to alter that choice in the middle of a course of treatment without full consultation between the members of the ECT team. Changes may happen inadvertently if the regular anaesthetist is unavailable.

Muscle relaxants

Muscle relaxants are used to ameliorate the convulsive muscle activity during stimulation and the subsequent seizure and reduce the risk of injury. In most cases it is not desirable to ablate all visible signs of muscle activity since this is a useful indicator of seizure induction. The duration of visible muscle activity should be recorded as a distinct parameter separate from any measured EEG activity. In cases where profound muscle relaxation is deemed necessary to protect the patient, the absence of visible clonic activity does not necessarily indicate failure to produce a seizure. This conclusion can be reached only if there is also no evidence of cerebral seizure activity (see Chapter 17).

An appropriate dose of muscle relaxant coupled with a suitable electrical stimulus should produce the classic, well-modified (bilateral) convulsion, but, as with the induction agent, subsequent doses should always be reviewed in the light of the patient's changing response to continued therapy.

Muscle relaxation is usually achieved with suxamethonium (0.5–1 mg/kg), but if this is contraindicated a short-acting non-depolarising agent can be used. A true rapid-sequence induction with cricoid pressure and endotracheal intubation should be reserved for those occasions when regurgitation of stomach contents remains a real risk despite the protective measures of antacid therapy and appropriate fasting. Suxamethonium remains the relaxant of first choice; it is given after loss of consciousness. The electrical stimulus should be applied only after fasciculations have ceased. Pseudocholinesterase deficiency, neuromuscular disease, the presence of cholinesterase inhibitors, a history of malignant hyperthermia, neuroleptic malignant syndrome, catatonia or major burns may preclude its use and suggest conversion to a non-depolarising agent.

Atracurium (0.3–0.5 mg/kg) or rocuronium (0.6–0.9 mg/kg) may be acceptable alternatives, although their relatively prolonged action may need to be actively reversed after treatment. Some authorities recommend the routine use of a neuromuscular nerve stimulator to ascertain both the adequacy of the block and its subsequent safe reversal. Sufficient time must be allowed for the onset of a non-depolarising block (Fredman *et al*, 1994).

Coexisting conditions such as severe cachexia, osteoporosis or skeletal injury may indicate the need to increase the dose of muscle relaxant.

The initial direct tetanic stimulation of the masseter by the electrodes should not be mistaken for inadequate muscle relaxation. It is this unavoidable maximal stimulation that presents the greatest danger to the patient's dentition and demands the prior positioning of a suitable bite block in all but the edentulous. Reusable bite blocks introduce the possibility of the transmission of infectious material between patients unless they are rigorously cleaned and sterilised. A tightly rolled and taped 4-inch swab can be used as a soft, cheap, effective and disposable bite block. To minimise the risk of damage to dentition, the lower jaw should be held firmly closed as the stimulus is applied.

Seizure induction

A period of hyperventilation (approximately 20 breaths) immediately before the application of the electrical stimulus has been shown to enhance seizure duration (Chater & Simpson, 1988).

A well-modified seizure will be manifest as minor tonic, followed by clonic activity of skeletal muscle, accompanied by a typical seizure pattern on EEG as described in Chapter 17. The absence of both is deemed a missed seizure.

During the clonic phase of the seizure, manual ventilation with 100% oxygen is quite easily achieved in most patients, and the measured oxygen saturation should never fall below 90%.

Missed seizures

Missed seizures may be due to insufficient stimulus intensity, excess dynamic impedance, premature stimulus termination, hypercarbia, dehydration or the effects of other treatment (e.g. benzodiazepines). The patient may develop a marked bradycardia, and atropine or glycopyrrolate should be available. After checking the electrode position, restimulation at a higher dose is possible, but a delay of at least 20 seconds should be incorporated to allow for the development of any delayed seizure. For future treatments a decrease in anaesthetic dose should be considered; U&Es should be checked and a change from a barbiturate induction to an alternative should be considered, as should benzodiazepine reversal, as discussed above.

One of the causes of missed or focal seizures is excess anaesthetic agent. Restimulation after a focal seizure is possible, but a delay of 45–90 seconds should be allowed for central repolarisation, after which, paradoxically, more anaesthetic may be needed.

Prolonged or tardive seizures

A prolonged seizure (duration > 2 minutes) and a tardive seizure (late return of seizure activity) are later complications, with the latter likely to occur in recovery. The principles of treatment are to maintain oxygenation and to monitor EEG activity; the anaesthetist should be prepared to abort the seizure with further doses of anaesthetic agents or benzodiazepines.

Record keeping and organisation

The doses of all anaesthetic agents used, the patient's response, and monitor recordings before and immediately after treatment and in recovery should be recorded and dated, and the records signed. Information pertinent to future treatments should also be noted.

With good patient preparation it will be rare that additional medication is needed. However, circumstances can arise when it may be necessary to modify unwanted autonomic, cardiovascular, respiratory or neurological effects and timely pharmacological intervention may reduce morbidity. The following additional agents need not be immediately available but it is suggested that they, or suitable alternatives, are accessible without undue delay: esmolol, adenosine, amiodarone, hydralazine, metaraminol, ephedrine, lidocaine, GTN spray, digoxin, verapamil, epinephrine, diphenhydramine, hydrocortisone, salbutamol, midazolam, flumazenil, frusemide, ondansetron, diclofenac, sodium citrate, neostigmine, glycopyrrolate, paracetamol and dantrolene sodium.

The risks of significant morbidity or mortality with patients properly prepared for ECT are low and compare favourably with those of minor (day-case type) surgery (Abrams, 1997). Patients who are perceived not to fall into this category (ASA grade III or above) should be treated in a specialised area and never in a remote location without critical-care backup.

Recovery area

This should be immediately accessible from the treatment area and be staffed by trained recovery personnel. The number of staff in the recovery area should exceed the number of unconscious patients by one.

Each first-stage recovery bay should be equipped with:

- oxygen supply (and spare), tubing, mask or nasal cannulae
- suction, with suitable cannulae/catheters
- pulse oximetry
- NIBP monitor or sphygmomanometer.

In addition, there should be access to electrocardiographic monitoring if necessary, and absorbent pillow protectors are useful.

The need to maintain a safe staff/patient ratio in the immediate recovery area means that the throughput of patients from the treatment area may need to be controlled. Post-treatment oxygen supplementation should be continued until pulse oximetry indicates that the patient can maintain a satisfactory SpO_2 on air (McCormick & Saunders, 1996).

The patient may be transferred to second-stage recovery once conscious, stable and able to maintain an airway.

Blood pressure and pulse oximeter readings should be continued and recorded during patient recovery. Patients should remain in the second-stage recovery area until they are haemodynamically stable. The presence of an escort with whom the patient is familiar can be very reassuring during the later stages of recovery, and can free the recovery staff to attend to subsequent patients.

Finally, the patient should walk, escorted, to sit in the final recovery lounge for a drink and a biscuit until deemed fit to return to home, the ward or day hospital. Written instructions covering the post-treatment period should be provided to new patients and their escort. A record should be kept of all personnel involved in the treatment episode and the anaesthetist must remain immediately available until the last patient is deemed fit for discharge.

References

Abrams, R. (1997) The mortality rate with ECT. *Convulsive Therapy*, **13**, 125–127.

Association of Anaesthetists of Great Britain and Ireland (1998) *The Anaesthesia Team*. London: AAGBI.

Association of Anaesthetists of Great Britain and Ireland (2000) *Recommendations for Standards of Monitoring During Anaesthesia and Recovery* (3rd edn). London: AAGBI.

Avramov, M. N., Husain, M. M. & White, P. F. (1995) Comparative effects of metho-hexitone, propofol and etomidate for ECT. *Anesthesia and Analgesia*, **81**, 596–602.

Bailine, S. H., Safferman, A., Vital-Herne, J., *et al* (1994) Flumazenil reversal of benzodiazepine-induced sedation for a patient with severe pre-ECT anxiety. *Convulsive Therapy*, **10**, 65–68.

Castelli, I., Steiner, L. A., Kaufmann, M. A., *et al* (1995) Comparative effects of esmolol and labetolol to attenuate hyperdynamic states after electroconvulsive therapy. *Anesthesia and Analgesia*, **80**, 557–561.

Chater, S. N., & Simpson, K. H. (1988) Effect of passive hyperventilation on seizure duration in patients undergoing ECT. *British Journal of Anaesthesia*, **60**, 70–73.

Diprose, P. & Pierce, J. M. T. (2001) CEPD reviews. *British Journal of Anaesthesia*, **1**, 166–170.

Fear, C. F., Littlejohns, S., Rouse, E., *et al* (1994) Propofol anaesthesia in electro-convulsive therapy. Reduced seizure duration may not be relevant. *British Journal of Psychiatry*, **165**, 506–509.

Fredman, B., Smith, I., d'Etienne, J., *et al* (1994) Use of muscle relaxants for electroconvulsive therapy: how much is enough? *Anesthesia and Analgesia*, **78**, 195–196.

Hanania, M. M. (1995) Flumazenil reversal of benzodiazepine sedation before electroconvulsive therapy. *Anesthesiology*, **82**, 321.

Kadar, A. G., Ing, C. H. & White, P. F. (2002) Anesthesia for electroconvulsive therapy in obese patients. *Anesthesia and Analgesia*, **94**, 360–361.

Kadoi, Y., Saito, S., Ide, M., *et al* (2003) The comparative effects of propofol versus thiopentone on left ventricular function during electroconvulsive therapy. *Anaesthesia and Intensive Care*, **31**, 172–175.

Kelly, K. G. & Zisselman, M. (2000) Update on electroconvulsive therapy (ECT) in older adults. *Journal of the American Geriatrics Society*, **48**, 560–566.

Mayur, P. M., Shree, R. S. & Gangadhar, B. N. (1998) Atropine pre-medication and the cardiovascular response to ECT. *British Journal of Anaesthesia*, **81**, 466–467.

McCormick, A. S. M. & Saunders, D. A. (1996) Oxygen saturation of patients recovering from electroconvulsive therapy. *Anaesthesia*, **51**, 702–704.

Pinski, S. L. & Trohman, R. G. (1995) Implantable cardioverter-defibrillators: implications for the nonelectrophysiologist. *Annals of Internal Medicine*, **122**, 770–777.

Pornnoppadol, C. & Isenberg, K. (1998) ECT with implantable cardioverter defibrillator. *Journal of ECT*, **14**, 124–126.

Rasmussen, K. G., Jarvis, M. R. & Zorumski, C. F. (1996) Ketamine anesthesia in electroconvulsive therapy. *Convulsive Therapy*, **12**, 217–223.

Rice, E. H., Sombrotto, L. B., Markowitz, J. C., *et al* (1994) Cardiovascular morbidity in high risk patients during ECT. *American Journal of Psychiatry*, **151**, 1637–1641.

Saklad, M. (1941) Grading of patients for surgical procedures. *Anesthesiology*, **2**, 281–284.

Simpson, K. & Lynch, L. (1998) Anaesthesia and ECT. *Anaesthesia*, **53**, 615–617.

Further reading

Ding, Z. & White, P. F. (2002) Anesthesia for electroconvulsive therapy. *Anesthesia and Analgesia*, **94**, 1351–1364.

Ishikawa, T., Kawahara, S., Saito, T., *et al* (2001) Anesthesia for electroconvulsive therapy during pregnancy – a case report. *Masui*, **50**, 991–997.

Mokriski, B. K., Nagle, S. E., Papuchis, G. C., *et al* (1992) Electroconvulsive therapy-induced cardiac arrhythmias during anesthesia with methohexital, thiamylal, or thiopental sodium. *Journal of Anesthesia*, **4**, 208–212.

CHAPTER 15

Prescribing

Allan I. F. Scott

The previous edition of the present book dealt separately with pre-scribing decisions presumed to be taken by the referring team and more technical details of treatment presumed to be decided by the staff of the ECT clinic. While there would be no bar to the referring team prescribing all aspects of treatment, this is unusual if the results of the nationwide audit in Scotland can be extrapolated to the rest of the UK (Freeman *et al*, 2000). The present chapter therefore follows the convention from the previous edition, and while this chapter deals with the prescription made by the referring team, Chapter 16 covers the practical details decided in the ECT clinic.

The referring team usually selects the electrode placement, and prescribes the frequency and total number of treatments. There is very little evidence about ECT technique in the treatment of mania (see Chapter 3), schizophrenia (see Chapter 4) and neuropsychiatric con-ditions (see Chapter 5); the present chapter concerns the available evidence that is from the treatment of depressive illness. It would be reasonable to apply the principles developed from the treatment of depressive illness in the treatment of these other conditions.

Electrode placement

The choice between unilateral and bilateral electrode placement remains controversial, but at least the results of the systematic review conducted by the UK ECT Review Group are now available to inform the choice (see Chapters 1 and 2). The results largely supported the recom-mendations in the previous edition that the bilateral placement was preferred when speed and/or completeness of recovery had priority, and that unilateral placement was preferred when minimising cognitive adverse effects had priority. Sufferers themselves may well be able and willing to express a view about the perceived severity of their illness, the need for urgent treatment, and a preference for a unilateral or bilateral electrode placement. This is particularly important in sufferers who have never before been treated with ECT and therefore have no personal experience to help balance the immediate benefits with longer-term risks such as distressing retrograde amnesia (see Chapter 1). What is clear is that no simple didactic statement can be made about the electrode placement of choice in all indications for ECT. The final selection of electrode placement ought to be the result of a balance of the estimated risks and benefits for the sufferer at a particular point in the illness, and informed, where possible, by the views of the sufferer.

In the Scottish audit of 1998/99, only 10 out of 717 patients were treated solely by unilateral ECT (Freeman *et al*, 2000). Many practitioners presumably remain sceptical about unilateral treatment because of earlier experiences of its limited efficacy, when it was given with inadequate electrical stimulation. While treatment with bilateral ECT retains an important place in treating patients who suffer severe or life-threatening illness and where the speed of improvement is critical, there are many other contemporary indications where the urgency of response is not critical (see Chapters 1 and 2). The guidance from the National Institute for Clinical Excellence (see Chapter 1) concluded that for too many sufferers the immediate benefit from ECT was outweighed by subsequent cognitive impairment attributed to ECT. When treatment is not urgent, an initial trial of unilateral ECT will significantly shift the cost–benefit balance because of the substantial reduction in the risk of severe or persistent retrograde amnesia (Lisanby *et al*, 2000). An increase in the use of unilateral ECT may be an important strategy to address the concerns of the NICE guidance.

When the initial prescription is of a unilateral electrode placement, it would be prudent to review this prescription after, say, the first four treatments. Clinical monitoring of symptoms and possible cognitive adverse effects is necessary in any case throughout treatment, and a lack of satisfactory improvement may lead to an increase in the electrical dose (see Chapter 16) or a switch to bilateral electrode placement if there had been no clinical improvement.

Choice of side in unilateral ECT

There is no evidence that the choice of side for unilateral ECT affects clinical efficacy, but treatment given over the cerebral hemisphere that is not dominant for language function is preferred because of its less noticeable cognitive effects. Unfortunately, there has not been a recent study that has assessed cognitive function in patients randomised to either dominant or non-dominant unilateral ECT with contemporary types of electrical stimulation, but older studies found that patients treated by non-dominant unilateral ECT regained orientation more quickly and experienced less severe impairment of verbal memory than patients treated with dominant unilateral ECT (see Daniel & Crovitz, 1983).

Handedness is related to cerebral dominance for language, but not exactly. In right-handed people, the vast majority will have dominant language function in the left cerebral hemisphere. In left-handed people, the relationship is more complicated: the majority will still have dominant language function in the left cerebral hemisphere, but in a minority neither cerebral hemisphere is dominant and in a further minority the right cerebral hemisphere is dominant.

The assessment of handedness should not just rest on the patient's preference for writing, and enquiry should be made about the preference for writing, throwing and using a tool (Pratt et al, 1971). The selection of right unilateral ECT is straightforward in patients who express a consistent preference for the right hand in all three tasks. Selection is more difficult in patients who have no consistent preference of hand and also for consistent left-handers. Bilateral ECT may be preferable, but an alternative strategy, rarely used, is to measure the time to recover after a unilateral treatment given over the right side and compare this with treatment given to the left side in the next treatment. Another test sensitive to cerebral dominance is the ability to name objects from an outline drawing (Pratt et al, 1971).

High-dose unilateral ECT

The most recent unresolved controversy is about whether or not unilateral ECT can be made just as efficacious as bilateral ECT by the use of a high electrical dose. There have been only two randomised controlled trials (RCTs) in which the two have been compared using electrical doses contingent on the known seizure threshold. In the first, unilateral ECT with a dose at six times the seizure threshold was compared with bilateral ECT given at a dose two-and-a-half times the seizure threshold (Sackeim et al, 2000). Immediately after the course of treatment, the proportion of patients who met a predetermined criterion of clinical response was identical in each arm (80%). The patients treated with bilateral ECT were slightly less depressed (approximately 2.5 points on the Hamilton Rating Scale for Depression), but this difference was not statistically significant. In the second, the dose given to patients treated with unilateral ECT was even higher (eight times the threshold) and compared with a lower dose of bilateral ECT (only one-and-a-half times the seizure threshold). McCall et al (2002) found that 60% of the patients treated with unilateral ECT and 73% of the patients treated with bilateral ECT met a predetermined criterion for clinical response immediately after the course of treatment. Patients treated with bilateral ECT were slightly less depressed (1.1 points on the Hamilton Rating Scale for Depression). Neither of these differences was statistically significant. The authors acknowledged that the modest number of included patients may have meant that the study lacked the statistical power to conclude confidently that the two treatments were of equal efficacy. Both studies reported that there were patients who did not recover with high-dose unilateral ECT, but who eventually recovered with supra-threshold bilateral treatment.

Recommendations

- Neither unilateral nor bilateral electrode placement is the treatment of choice in all indications for ECT (see below).
- The selection of electrode placement should, where possible, be part of the process of informed consent for ECT.
- Where the rate of clinical improvement and completeness of response have priority, bilateral placement is preferable.
- Where minimising the cognitive adverse effects has priority, unilateral placement is preferable. This may be particularly relevant in neuropsychiatric conditions such as Parkinson's disease (see Chapter 5).
- Bilateral electrode placement will also be preferred:
  - where the index episode of illness or an earlier episode of illness had not been treated adequately by unilateral ECT
  - where determining cerebral dominance is difficult
  - in the treatment of mania, where the optimal technique for the use of unilateral ECT has not been established (see Chapter 3).
- Unilateral electrode placement will also be preferred:
  - where the rate of clinical improvement is not critical
  - where there is a history of recovery with unilateral ECT.
- Right unilateral ECT is preferred in people who are consistently right-handed.
- In left-handed people or where cerebral dominance is hard to decide,
  - bilateral electrode placement may be preferred
  - alternatively, an empirical trial may be made when the time to recover orientation is compared between right- and left-sided treatment given at consecutive treatment sessions under standard conditions.

Frequency of treatments

Bilateral ECT

The evidence from RCTs on the relationship between the efficacy of ECT and the frequency of treatment concerned mainly treatment with bilateral ECT, and was assessed by the UK ECT Review Group (see

Chapter 2). There was no evidence that bilateral ECT given three times each week was more efficacious than treatment twice a week as measured by reduction in depressive symptoms after a complete course of treatment. A meta-analysis of the comparative effects on cognitive function was not possible, but individual RCTs show clearly that the higher frequency of treatment causes more cognitive adverse effects (Shapira *et al*, 1998).

Some practitioners prescribe bilateral ECT three times in the first week in the emergency treatment of severe depressive illness (see Chapter 2), presumably on the assumption that this will increase the rate of improvement. This assumption has never been empirically tested, and is open to question (see Shapira *et al*, 1998). The greatest reduction in depressive symptoms occurs with the first bilateral administration of ECT and there is no difference in the reduction in depressive symptoms between twice and thrice weekly ECT after three administrations; the advantage in favour of thrice weekly treatment is seen only after four treatments and becomes clinically meaningful only after five treatments. It is not certain that 1 week of thrice weekly treatment would be sufficient to initiate this course of more rapid clinical improvement.

In contrast, it has been shown that high-dose bilateral ECT (two-and-a-half times the seizure threshold) leads to greater clinical improvement over the first six treatments than threshold bilateral ECT (Sackeim *et al*, 1993). The need for emergency treatment may therefore be an indication for bilateral ECT at a dose at the upper end of the recommended range; this would be at the cost of more pronounced cognitive adverse effects (Sackeim *et al*, 1993; see also Chapters 2 and 16).

Unilateral ECT

There has been only one small RCT that compared the efficacy and cognitive adverse effects of unilateral ECT given two or three times per week (McAllister *et al*, 1987). Unfortunately, the study was conducted at a time when the importance of electrical dose was not fully appreciated, and no attempt was made to relate electrical doses to seizure threshold; it is likely that treatment was akin to low-dose unilateral ECT. There was no suggestion that depressive symptoms measured by the Hamilton Rating Scale for Depression fell more quickly with three treatments per week over the first two weeks. Interestingly, measurements of new learning and visual–motor problem solving actually improved over the course of ECT with treatment both twice and three times per week (see also Chapter 16); improvement was less marked in patients treated three times per week. This lack of evidence may not be of great importance because unilateral electrode placement is preferred when the rate of clinical improvement is not critical. It may become clinically important in the emergency treatment of severe depressive illness where the sufferer elects to be treated by unilateral ECT, or where there is a history of intolerable cognitive adverse effects with bilateral ECT. This is an indication for the use of an electrical dose at the upper end of the recommended range from the first treatment in a course (see Chapter 16) because it has been shown that higher doses in right unilateral ECT lead to greater clinical improvement over the first six treatments (Sackeim *et al*, 2000).

Lower-frequency treatment

The frequency of treatment may be reduced below twice per week to, say, weekly to reduce treatment-emergent cognitive adverse effects, especially as the end-point of a course of treatment is approached.

Recommendations

- In bilateral ECT:
  - the optimal frequency is twice per week
  - the frequency may be reduced to, say, weekly in the management of treatment-emergent cognitive adverse effects
  - administration three times per week does not increase the likelihood of eventual recovery, but leads to a more rapid reduction in depressive symptoms over a course of treatment at the cost of more pronounced cognitive adverse effects – it would therefore be justified only in severe, life-threatening illnesses and only as long as the illness remained severe and/ or life-threatening (an alternative evidence-based strategy would be to ensure that the initial dose in twice weekly treatment is 50–100% above the seizure threshold – see Chapters 2 and 16).
- In unilateral ECT:
  - the optimal frequency is probably twice per week
  - there is no evidence that administering treatment three times per week leads to more rapid reduction in symptoms (an alternative evidence-based strategy would be to ensure that the initial dose is 300–500% above the seizure threshold – see Chapter 16).

Number of treatments

A set number of treatments should not be prescribed at the start of a course of ECT. The patient should be assessed after each treatment to see if further treatments are necessary. It was noted above that the most marked reduction in symptoms is after the first bilateral administration of ECT, and some patients respond dramatically to the few treatments. Other patients may require 12 or more treatments first.

The most difficult clinical decision remains at what stage to abandon ECT if it is proving ineffective. There has been some work in this area, at least in the treatment of depressive illness with supra-threshold bilateral ECT. The extent of clinical improvement over the first few treatments is closely correlated with the extent of eventual improvement (see Rodger *et al*, 1994; Segman *et al*, 1995). If no clinical improvement at all has been seen over the first six bilateral treatments, then it is highly unlikely that more treatments will bring about either significant clinical improvement or eventual recovery (Segman *et al*, 1995). The previous edition of this handbook suggested, only as a guideline, that it may be reasonable to give up to 12 treatments to patients who display definite but slight or temporary improvement over the first few treatments; this turned out to be entirely compatible with the observation that a small but significant minority of depressed patients respond fully to treatments beyond the eighth of a course, having shown only modest improvement with earlier treatments (Segman *et al*, 1995). This observation is also compatible with the results of the nationwide Scottish audit (Freeman *et al*, 2000).

There has never been an RCT of the treatment of patients with depression who have failed to improve sufficiently with right unilateral ECT, but patients who subsequently recover with bilateral ECT require a similar number of treatments to those initially treated from the outset with bilateral ECT. It would seem reasonable to discount the previous unilateral treatments in patients who have switched from unsuccessful unilateral treatment, and to assess their need for treatment afresh using the same principles as for bilateral ECT.

Recommendations

- It is not possible to predict reliably how many treatments will be required in a course of ECT. A set course of treatments should therefore not be prescribed.
- The need for further treatment should be assessed after each individual treatment.
- If no clinical improvement at all is seen after six properly given bilateral treatments, then the course should be abandoned.
- It may be worth continuing up to 12 bilateral treatments before abandoning ECT in patients who have shown definite but slight or temporary improvement with early treatments.
- There are some patients with depression who do not respond to high-dose right unilateral ECT, but who subsequently respond to bilateral ECT. The ineffective unilateral treatments should be disregarded in the assessment of need for further bilateral treatments.

References

Daniel, W. F. & Crovitz, H. F. (1983) Acute memory impairment following electro-convulsive therapy, 2: effects of electrode placement. *Acta Psychiatrica Scandinavica*, **67**, 57–68.

Freeman, C. P. L., Hendry, J. & Fergusson, G. (2000) *National Audit of Electroconvulsive Therapy in Scotland. Final Report.* Available at www.sean.org.uk/report/report00.php.

Lisanby, S. H., Maddox, J. H., Prudic, J., et al (2000) The effects of electroconvulsive therapy on memory of autobiographical and public events. *Archives of General Psychiatry*, **57**, 581–590.

McAllister, D. A., Perri, M. G., Jordan, R. C., et al (1987) Effects of ECT given two vs. three times weekly. *Psychiatry Research*, **21**, 63–69.

McCall, W. V., Dunn, A., Rosenquist, P. B., et al (2002) Markedly suprathreshold right unilateral ECT versus minimally suprathreshold bilateral ECT: antidepressant and memory effects. *Journal of ECT*, **18**, 126–129.

Pratt, R. T. C., Warrington, E. K. & Halliday, A. M. (1971) Unilateral ECT as a test for cerebral dominance, with a strategy for treating left-handers. *British Journal of Psychiatry*, **119**, 79–83.

Rodger, C. R., Scott, A. I. & Whalley, L. J. (1994) Is there a delay in the onset of the antidepressant effect of electroconvulsive therapy? *British Journal of Psychiatry*, **164**, 106–109.

Sackeim, H. A., Prudic, J., Devanand, D. P., et al (1993) Effects of stimulus intensity and electrode placement on the efficacy and cognitive effects of electroconvulsive therapy. *New England Journal of Medicine*, **328**, 839–846.

Sackeim, H. A., Prudic, J., Devanand, D. P., et al (2000) A prospective, randomised, double-blind comparison of bilateral and right unilateral electroconvulsive therapy at different stimulus intensity. *Archives of General Psychiatry*, **57**, 425–434.

Segman, R. H., Shapira, B., Gorfin, M., et al (1995) Onset and time course of antidepressant action: psychopharmacological implications of a controlled trial of electroconvulsive therapy. *Psychopharmacology*, **119**, 440–448.

Shapira, B., Tubi, N., Drexler, H., et al (1998) Cost and benefit in the choice of ECT schedule. Twice versus three times weekly ECT. *British Journal of Psychiatry*, **172**, 44–48.

CHAPTER 16

Practical administration of ECT

Allan I. F. Scott

This chapter concerns the practical and technical details of treatment presumed to be decided by the staff of the ECT clinic. Chapter 15 suggested that an increase in the use of unilateral ECT by prescribers may be an important strategy to address the concerns of the guidance from the National Institute for Clinical Excellence (NICE) discussed in Chapter 1. ECT practitioners will be familiar with the observation that most developments of ECT practice have been driven not by the need to make ECT more efficacious but to reduce its adverse effects; this chapter recommends important changes to how ECT is administered to address the same concerns.

The aim of ECT

The aim of ECT is to induce generalised cerebral seizure activity of a type that is associated with a tonic–clonic or grand mal convulsion, and to do so with an electrical dose that is sufficiently above the seizure threshold to maximise the clinical efficacy of treatment, but not so high that it needlessly contributes to the cognitive effects of treatment. (The necessary seizure activity is described and illustrated in detail in Chapter 17.)

The ECT machine

It is already a recommendation that treatment is given by an ECT machine that delivers a measured dose of electrical charge, that is, a constant-current stimulus, and that this be delivered by a train of brief pulses, usually around 1 ms in length. The machine must also be able to deliver a wide range of electrical dose, usually measured in units of electrical charge (usually stated as millicoulombs); this would normally be from 25–50 mC up to 750–800 mC. This is necessary because a wide range of seizure threshold is observed among patients of differing age and gender, and where many may be taking psychotropic drugs that both inhibit and promote the induction of cerebral seizure. When a machine needs to be replaced, it would be desirable to purchase a machine with a higher output, able to provide unilateral treatment with doses up to six times the initial seizure threshold. This may require a machine with an output of up to 1000 mC.

The previous edition (published in 1995) of the present work devoted some space to describing the different types of electrical waveform used by different machines and how each parameter of the waveform might be altered to adjust the administered electrical dose. Nearly all ECT machines bought in the UK now use a single dial to adjust the electrical dose; most practitioners do not therefore have the ability to adjust individual parameters of the electrical stimulus – unless a commercial machine is specially modified. There is an important research interest in how adjustments in the width of the brief pulses and their frequency affect the ease of induction, clinical efficacy and cognitive effects of treatment; the interested reader is directed to a specialist textbook (for example, Abrams, 2002) or a specialist journal such as the *Journal of ECT*. Commercial manufacturers of ECT machines available in the UK are listed in Appendix X.

Recommendations

- ECT is administered by a constant-current, brief-pulse ECT machine that is able to deliver a wide range of electrical dose, that is, 25–50 mC up to 750–800 mC.
- It is recommended that new machines deliver a range of dose from 25 to 1000 mC.

Electrode placement

Bilateral ECT

The traditional positioning for the electrodes in bilateral ECT is illustrated in Figure 16.1 (left). The centre of the electrode should be 4 cm above, and perpendicular to, the mid-point of a line between the lateral angle of the eye and the external auditory meatus. One electrode is applied thus to each side of the head, and this positioning is referred to as bi-temporal ECT. (Some writers refer to bi-frontotemporal ECT.) These are the recommended positions for the electrodes in bilateral ECT because this has become the standard positioning, and it cannot be assumed that the latest research findings can be extrapolated to other positionings in bilateral ECT.

There have been other experimental positionings for the electrodes in bilateral ECT. Bi-frontal ECT, where the electrodes were spaced only

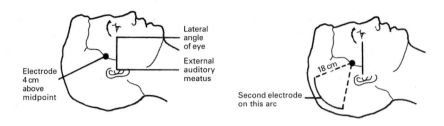

Figure 16.1 The temporal positioning (left) and temporoparietal or d'Elia positioning (right) of electrodes.

about 5 cm (2 inches) apart and each about 5 cm above the bridge of the nose, was abandoned because of the shunting of electrical current between the electrodes. A more recent modification where the electrodes were applied further apart has been investigated because its advocates suggested that it might be as efficacious as traditional bilateral ECT, but with a lower risk of cognitive adverse effects. The UK ECT Review Group (2003) found no significant difference between traditional bilateral ECT and wide-spaced bi-frontal ECT either in clinical efficacy or in cognitive adverse effects; however, the fairest conclusion may be that the relatively small number of included patients in the Review Group's meta-analysis meant that it lacked the statistical power for a meaningful comparison.

Unilateral ECT

The traditional position of the electrodes in unilateral ECT is illustrated in Figure 16.1 (right). This positioning is usually referred to as the temporoparietal or d'Elia position, in which one electrode is in the same position as in traditional bilateral ECT and the other applied over the parietal surface of the scalp. The exact position on the parietal arc is not crucial; the aims are to maximise the distance between the electrodes to reduce shunting of electrical current and to choose a site on the arc where the electrode can be applied firmly and flat against the scalp. Unilateral ECT is usually applied over the non-dominant hemisphere, which is the right side of the head in most people (see Chapter 15). These are the recommended positions in unilateral ECT because this had become the standard, and it cannot be assumed that the latest research findings can be extrapolated to other positionings.

It is sometimes written that unilateral ECT is the more difficult treatment to administer. This can be so if the treating doctor is left alone to position and then support the patient's head, and then apply the electrodes. Unilateral ECT can be administered effectively when it is viewed as a shared responsibility of the ECT clinic team. Some anaesthetists routinely ask patients to turn on to their left sides before the induction of anaesthesia. The assistance of a nurse or a member of the anaesthetic staff is essential to undertake the tasks of turning the patient's head to make available the parietal aspect of the scalp and to support the head adequately by a pillow or similar.

Recommendations

- In bilateral ECT, the recommended position of the electrodes is the bi-temporal positioning, as illustrated in Figure 16.1 (left).
- In unilateral ECT, the recommended position of the electrodes is the temporo-parietal or d'Elia positioning, as illustrated in Figure 16.1 (right).

Stimulus dosing

The most important decision taken by the ECT practitioner in the clinic is the selection of the electrical dose for the individual patient, what is now referred to as stimulus dosing. The recent NICE guidance (see Chapter 1) concluded that for some patients the distress caused by persistent or severe memory problems subsequently attributed to ECT outweigh the original clinical benefit. This chapter will recommend changes to practice to address this concern and some space will be devoted to the rationale behind them.

Practical administration and cognitive effects

British psychiatry can be commended for its reappraisal of ECT, which included several randomised comparisons of active treatment with sham ECT (UK ECT Review Group, 2003). The primary aim of these studies was to reassess the clinical efficacy of ECT. It is only with hindsight that it is appreciated how an opportunity was missed systematically to assess treatment-emergent adverse effects, in a comparison of real and sham ECT. None of these randomised controlled trials included, for example, any bedside tests of cognitive function. Many British ECT practitioners believed that the introduction of modern brief-pulse ECT machines meant that few patients experienced profound or troublesome cognitive adverse effects, even when bilateral ECT was used (Lock, 1995). The reasons why this genuinely held view may have evolved have been discussed elsewhere (Rose *et al*, 2003). ECT practitioners of the time may not have been so familiar with contemporaneous studies of the neurobiology of ECT. These found that ECT technique continued to have an important effect on the cognitive effects of treatment, and in particular the use of a bilateral electrode placement (Sackeim *et al*, 1986; Scott *et al*, 1990).

The effects of ECT technique on cognition in contemporary practice can be illustrated by examination of the raw data from one of the recent studies from the USA (Sackeim *et al*, 2000); these findings are consistent with those from other studies. On average, patients with depression treated with low-dose right unilateral ECT become reorientated within 20 minutes of treatment; the same is true for patients treated with a moderate dose, that is, two-and-a-half times the seizure threshold. Patients treated with high-dose right unilateral ECT, that is, six times the seizure threshold, take about 30 minutes to become reorientated. In contrast, patients treated with bilateral ECT, with a dose two-and-a-half times the seizure threshold, take 15 minutes longer yet to become reorientated – 45 minutes. The risk of prolonged disorientation is less than 1% for low-dose and moderate-dose unilateral ECT; about 2% for high-dose unilateral dose ECT; but 13% for bilateral ECT. The important effect of bilateral electrode placement is emphasised when it is noted that the electrical dose in high-dose right unilateral ECT was more than 100 mC (or 43%) greater than that used in bilateral ECT, yet these patients became reorientated more quickly than those treated by bilateral ECT. Even when bilateral ECT is given at a dose just above the seizure threshold, patients take, on average, 40 minutes to become reorientated, and 9% experience prolonged disorientation after at least one treatment in a course (Sackeim *et al*, 1993).

The problem for the ECT practitioner is that there is insufficient knowledge to allow a prediction of who among the patients now treated with ECT will later complain of the distressing memory problems that undo the clinical benefit of treatment; indeed, most patients included in contemporary ECT research report that their memory improved over treatment, presumably as their depressed mood lifted. It has not been shown conclusively that the measurable acute cognitive effects of ECT reliably predict the later risk of distressing memory problems attributed to ECT, but there is preliminary evidence that the duration of post-ECT disorientation correlates with measurable retrograde amnesia 2 months after treatment (Sobin *et al*, 1995). The evidence is sparse, but it would seem reasonable that the ECT practitioner do all he or she can to reduce the acute cognitive effects of ECT that must affect the patient's experience of treatment and that may be warning signs that the patient is at risk of severe or persistent memory problems. This may also be an important strategy to address the concerns of the NICE guidance.

Seizure threshold

The minimum electrical dose to induce the necessary generalised cerebral seizure activity is referred to as the seizure threshold. Electrical waveforms vary in the efficiency with which they induce seizures, and a reported seizure threshold is meaningful only when related to a particular ECT machine. The seizure threshold is also affected by factors that contribute to the electrical impedance, factors that affect the excitability of cerebral neurons, and ECT technique; in particular, initial seizure thresholds with bilateral placement are at least 40% higher than with unilateral placement, and it may therefore be helpful to consider the two techniques separately.

A recent collaborative study found that more than 40% of patients had an initial seizure threshold of less than 50 mC with a unilateral electrode placement (Boylan *et al*, 2000). (Many British ECT practitioners will be familiar with the Ectron series of ECT machines, the latest of which can deliver a minimum electrical dose of 50 mC; this study did not use an Ectron ECT machine, but suggested that a substantial proportion of patients have a low initial seizure threshold in the contemporary practice of unilateral ECT.) For bilateral ECT, the proportion of patients with an initial seizure threshold less than 50 mC is smaller, but not insignificant; it is 7% in the author's experience with an Ectron ECT machine (Scott & Dykes, 1999), almost identical to the proportion in a study from the USA (Sackeim *et al*, 1991). The vast majority of patients will have an initial seizure threshold of less than 200 mC, with either electrode placement. The proportion of patients who have an unusually high seizure threshold is debated and variation among clinics is likely to reflect differences between them in ECT and anaesthetic technique, as well as differences in the definition of the necessary seizure activity. Whatever the absolute proportion, the ECT practitioner will occasionally encounter patients with unusually high initial seizure thresholds, for example a bald, dehydrated, elderly man who is prescribed an anti-epileptic drug for mood stabilisation and who requires a larger than usual dose of induction agent because of severe agitation. In the management of such patients, it is important to try to modify factors that may reduce the seizure threshold to the more orthodox range – especially if the induction of the necessary cerebral seizure activity is problematic (see Chapters 12 and 14, and below).

Clinical relevance

The clinical relevance of the seizure threshold is becoming clearer. It was illustrated above how the acute cognitive effects of right unilateral ECT are positively correlated with the electrical dose when expressed as a multiple of the seizure threshold. It was noted in Chapter 15 that the rate of improvement in depressive symptoms over a course of unilateral ECT is likewise correlated with electrical dose when expressed as a multiple of the seizure threshold. It is shown below that the probability of clinical remission after a course of unilateral ECT is also related to electrical dose expressed in the same way. The importance of the electrical dose is not so great with bilateral ECT; nevertheless, the electrical dose expressed as a multiple of the seizure threshold is still correlated with the rate of improvement over the first six treatments (Sackeim *et al*, 1993), which is consistent with older studies that found that high-dose bilateral ECT accelerates the rate of clinical improvement (see Robin & De Tissera, 1982). The effect of electrical dose on the acute cognitive sequelae of bilateral ECT is much less striking than its effect in unilateral ECT, but the range of electrical dose that has been assessed systematically is much less for bilateral ECT; it may be important to recall that very high-dose bilateral ECT had already been shown to cause more anterograde and retrograde amnesia than any other ECT technique (Weiner *et al*, 1986).

The individual patient

If the electrical dose expressed as a multiple of the seizure threshold contributes both to efficacy and cognitive effects, and the initial seizure threshold varies substantially among patients, then it follows that the electrical dose must vary to suit the needs of the individual patient. This is an explicit and important change from the practice recommended in the previous (1995) edition of the present work, in which it was stated that it may be acceptable to select a dose that is known to be appropriate for the majority, that is, 80% or more of similar patients. It was observed, without comment, that many British ECT clinics gave bilateral ECT with a standard or fixed dose for all patients at the first treatment. Such a treatment policy for bilateral ECT can no longer pass without comment if the concerns of the NICE guidance are to be heeded. That edition did acknowledge that the main disadvantage of this fixed-dose policy was that the ECT practitioner did not know by how much the dose exceeded the seizure threshold in an individual patient. A standard fixed dose chosen to be high enough to ensure that most patients experience the necessary generalised cerebral seizure activity would be several times the initial seizure threshold for those patients with a seizure threshold less than 50 mC. Such a dose would contribute to acute and longer-term cognitive effects of treatment, without any commensurate effect on clinical efficacy (Weiner *et al*, 1986).

The initial seizure threshold cannot be predicted accurately for individual patients based on demographic or clinical features (see Boylan *et al*, 2000). On average, old men have higher initial seizure thresholds than, say, young women; but when tabulated raw data are reported, it can be seen that some old men have initial seizure thresholds as low as young women (Scott & Dykes, 1999; Chung & Wong, 2001). What this means for the ECT practitioner is that the only reliable way to identify patients with a low seizure threshold is to give a low electrical dose initially at the first treatment, to establish whether or not it is sufficient to induce the necessary seizure activity. In the general case, it may be reasonable to start at 50 mC, but it may be desirable to start with only 25 mC in special populations such as young people or patients prescribed psychotropic drugs known to lower the seizure threshold (see Chapter 12). If the necessary cerebral seizure is induced, then the initial seizure threshold has been established as 50 mC. If a seizure is not induced, then the ECT practitioner has at least established that the initial seizure threshold is above 50 mC; options for the second stimulation in this case are discussed below.

The Special Committee appreciated that some UK ECT clinics will have no experience in the empirical measurement of the seizure threshold, and that a recommendation for the introduction of this technique will have significant training and organisational implications. The priority is to avoid the scenario where a patient with a low seizure threshold receives an electrical dose many times his or her seizure threshold, particularly in bilateral ECT. While staff are being trained and gaining experience, it may therefore be a sufficient interim recommendation that clinics routinely identify those patients with a low seizure threshold. The routine use of an initial low electrical dose as described above would achieve this. If the necessary seizure is not induced, clinics with expertise in the empirical measurement of seizure threshold may go on by repeated stimulation to measure the seizure threshold, whereas clinics with less experience may use an estimate of the seizure threshold once the possibility of a low threshold has been excluded; the estimate may be taken from one of the commercially available schedules and the clinic's dosing strategy would then be applied to this estimate (see below).

Bilateral ECT – treatment to save life

When the ECT practitioner sets out to measure the seizure threshold, the aim is to use the minimum electrical dose to induce a seizure. This is therefore treatment at or just above the seizure threshold. This is not desirable when bilateral ECT is being given as emergency treatment to save life. The rate of clinical improvement is paramount here, and an initial dose 50–100% above the seizure threshold would be better (see Chapters 2 and 15). When bilateral ECT is potentially life-saving, it may be preferable to forego empirical measurement of the seizure threshold; the initial seizure threshold may instead be estimated and then the initial electrical dose would be 50–100% above this estimated value of the seizure threshold. Such treatment could be justified only while the illness is severe or life-threatening, and the routine empirical measurement could be made once the patient's condition had started to improve.

Unilateral ECT

There is still an understandable debate about whether or not empirical measurement of the seizure threshold is necessary for patients pre-scribed unilateral ECT. The arguments in favour of giving an initial dose several times the estimated seizure threshold are that such stimulation accelerates the clinical improvement and maximizes final efficacy, and that the patients do not run the same risk of troublesome cognitive adverse effects as when a bilateral electrode placement is used. A note of caution must be added: very high-dose right unilateral ECT may need to be given with the same caution as bilateral ECT because it has been shown that increasing the electrical dose from two-and-a-half times the seizure threshold to 8–12 times the seizure threshold has a greater impact on the acute cognitive effects of treatment than it does on antidepressant efficacy (McCall *et al*, 2000); moreover, a recent report failed to find any advantage for very high-dose unilateral ECT, that is, eight times the seizure threshold, over bilateral ECT in terms of cognitive adverse effects (McCall *et al*, 2002). This topic clearly merits further study. It may be reasonable in the meantime to forego empirical measurement of the seizure threshold and to estimate it when the aim is to give right unilateral ECT at a dose up to two or three times the seizure threshold. It may be better empirically to measure the seizure threshold when the aim is to give right unilateral ECT with higher doses, the only exception being where ECT is prescribed to save life, when an estimate of the seizure threshold could be used until the patient's condition had started to improve and then the routine empirical measurement could be made.

Recommendations

- Stimulus dosing, that is, the selection of electrical dose for an individual patient, is contingent upon the patient's seizure threshold.
- The initial seizure threshold cannot be reliably predicted for individual patients based on demographic or clinical features. Empirical measurement is the best available means of establishing the initial seizure threshold.
- The routine empirical measurement of the initial seizure threshold would be good practice in non-urgent treatment. The Special Committee accepts that some ECT clinics will have no experience of this technique, and as an interim step may prefer to develop experience by routinely identifying patients with a low initial seizure threshold by using a low electrical dose (25–50 mC) as the first stimulation at the first treatment.
- The exception may be in the management of life-threatening illness, where the rate of clinical improvement is critical and the

use of a threshold dose is undesirable; it would be better to estimate the seizure threshold using one of the commercially available schedules and use this estimate to calculate the treatment dose as per the clinic's dosing strategy (see below). The empirical measurement could be held over until the emergency is passing, later in the course of treatment.

- In bilateral ECT:
  - the use of a fixed or standard electrical dose is no longer acceptable, and one of the empirical techniques must be used in non-urgent treatments.
- In unilateral ECT:
  - there is still an understandable debate about the need to measure the seizure threshold
  - empirical measurement of the initial seizure threshold may not be crucial for electrical doses intended to be only two or three times the seizure threshold
  - when the intention is to use higher electrical doses, say, doses of three or four times the seizure threshold and above, it would be good practice to use one of the empirical techniques.

Dosing strategy

The effect of the electrical dose was considered by the UK ECT Review Group and the findings were discussed in Chapter 2. The evidence to show that the electrical dose affects the rate of clinical improvement over the first six treatments has been discussed above. A summary of the impact of electrical dose on final outcome is given here (and see Sackeim *et al*, 1993, 2000).

A proportion, but clearly a minority, of patients with depression will recover with moderate-dose unilateral ECT, that is, unilateral ECT given at a dose two-and-a-half times the seizure threshold. The majority of patients will recover with treatment given at a dose six times the seizure threshold, but at the cost of more pronounced adverse cognitive effects. One reasonable approach therefore may be to start the course of unilateral ECT at a dose about three times the seizure threshold, but be prepared to increase the dose to up to six times the seizure threshold in the absence of significant clinical improvement.

The majority of patients with depression will recover with bilateral ECT even if it is given at an electrical dose just above the seizure threshold. The clinical efficacy of ECT in depressive illness treated by bilateral ECT has been systematically evaluated only to a dose of 150 per cent above (i.e. two-and-a-half times) the seizure threshold. The research to date has not found an increase in the efficacy of bilateral ECT with higher doses. This may be only because the research so far has lacked the statistical power to conclude confidently that higher-dose bilateral ECT is no more efficacious than threshold treatment, but it is consistent with older studies (Weiner *et al*, 1986). It may be reasonable to start the course with a treatment dose 50% above (i.e. one-and-a-half times) the initial seizure threshold. The exception may be in the emergency treatment of life-threatening illness, when an initial dose 50–100% above the initial seizure threshold would be better (see Chapters 2 and 15). It would be reasonable gradually to increase the dose up to 150% above (i.e. two-and-a-half times) the seizure threshold if clinical improvement is inadequate.

There has been no systematic research on electrical doses above two-and-a-half times the seizure threshold, although some ECT researchers have suggested the use of higher doses than this in patients with depression who are still severely unwell after unsuccessful treatment with orthodox bilateral ECT. This would require more intensive research study before it could be recommended. There has never been a randomised controlled trial of the management of patients who had failed to improve substantially, if at all, with ECT, but there are alternative strategies (see Chapter 12).

Recommendations

- In unilateral ECT:
  - the initial electrical dose should be at least 200% above (i.e. three times) the initial seizure threshold
  - if clinical improvement is definite but slight or temporary after four to six treatments, then doses up to 500% above (i.e. six times) the seizure threshold are indicated.
- In bilateral ECT:
  - the initial electrical dose should be at least 50% above (i.e. one-and-a-half times) the initial seizure threshold
  - where emergency treatment is required to save life, the initial electrical dose should be at least 50–100% above the initial seizure threshold
  - if clinical improvement is inadequate after four to six treat-ments, then doses up to 150% above (i.e. two-and-a-half times) the seizure threshold are indicated.

Dose adjustments during the course of treatment

The seizure threshold may, but not inevitably, rise over the course of treatment. Ideally, the dose would rise *pari passu* with any rise in the seizure threshold to maintain the dosing strategy (see above). An early study found that the seizure threshold increased about 80% in bilateral ECT and 40% in unilateral ECT over a course of treatment (Sackeim *et al*, 1991). Recent studies found increases of only 25–40% for bilateral ECT (see Scott & Boddy, 2000). It was noted above that many factors affect the seizure threshold and to these can be added the prescription and technique of ECT when one considers how the initial seizure threshold may change over a course of treatment. It may be that the average change is not a useful statistic, and the ECT practitioner may be better guided by the advice that the initial seizure threshold changes only in a proportion of patients and, when this happens, the extent of the increase may vary widely, from a modest increase to two or more times the original threshold.

A rise in the seizure threshold may be obvious because an electrical dose that originally induced the necessary seizure fails to do so later in the course of treatment – the so-called missed seizure (see below). This is unlikely to happen with the dosing strategy for unilateral ECT recommended above, and in any case smaller rises in seizure threshold will not be so obvious. The previous edition of this handbook suggested that this may be apparent to the ECT practitioner because of a progressive shortening in the length of convulsions or seizures over the course of treatment. Unfortunately, further research found that there was only a modest correlation between the change in the length of convulsions and the change in the seizure threshold (Scott & Boddy, 2000). The ECT practitioner should still consider that the seizure threshold is rising when faced with such progressive shortening by checking the patient's clinical improvement; if this is satisfactory, then it is not necessary to increase the dose. If clinical improvement is absent or inadequate, then an increase in electrical dose is indicated, irrespective of the length of the convulsions. The monitoring of seizure activity by electroencephalogram (EEG) may contribute to the assessment for dose adjustments (see Chapter 17).

Significant cognitive adverse effects such as prolonged disorientation after treatment would be an indication to reduce the electrical dose. (Inadequate clinical improvement and treatment-emergent cognitive adverse effects will also affect the choice of electrode placement – see Chapter 15).

Recommendations

- Clinical monitoring is the best guide to what, if any, adjustment to the electrical dose is required over a course of treatment: absent or inadequate clinical improvement indicates a need for a higher electrical dose, while the emergence of significant cognitive adverse effects indicates that a lower electrical dose should be used.
- Clinical monitoring may also affect the choice of electrode placement (see Chapter 15).

Missed seizures

If the necessary cerebral seizure activity has not been induced, then the aim of ECT has not been achieved (see Chapter 17 for the necessary monitoring). The ECT practitioner must restimulate the patient while he or she is still unconscious – otherwise the treatment session will have no therapeutic benefit. There is sometimes a latent period between the end of electrical stimulation and the clear-cut induction of cerebral seizure activity or a tonic–clonic convulsion. It is advisable to wait 20 seconds before restimulation, to exclude this possibility. A higher electrical dose will be required in the restimulation, but how much higher will depend on the aim of restimulation. The ECT practitioner may wish to establish the new seizure threshold, in which case stimulation with a dose only slightly higher is indicated, that is, 25–50 mC higher; if this slightly higher dose induces the necessary seizure activity, then the ECT practitioner will have learned that the new seizure threshold lies between the first dose (which did not induce a seizure) and the second, higher dose (which did). If the patient returns to the clinic for another treatment, then this new value for the seizure threshold can be used to calculate the treatment dose as per the clinic's dosing strategy.

When the ECT practitioner sets out to establish the seizure threshold, the aim is to use an electrical dose at or just above the patient's seizure threshold. The use of such a threshold dose will not be desirable when ECT is being used to treat a life-threatening illness because threshold ECT will not maximise the rate of clinical improvement. If a missed seizure has been identified and the illness is still life-threatening, then it would be better to restimulate the patient with a dose that will maximise the rate of clinical improvement. Instead of restimulation with a slightly higher dose, it may be better to estimate that the new seizure threshold is 25–50 mC higher and to use this estimate in the calculation of the treatment dose, as per the clinic's dosing strategy; for example, in the use of bilateral ECT for emergency treatment, the dose for restimulation would be 50–100% above the new estimated seizure threshold.

A rise in the patient's seizure threshold is only one of the possible explanations of a missed seizure. After successful restimulation, it is important to consider other causes of the missed seizure. The prescribed dose may not actually have been delivered because of some technical or operational problem. Consultation with the anaesthetist is necessary to review whether or not any change to anaesthetic technique may have contributed; a common reason for difficulty in the induction of cerebral seizure activity is the administration of an excessively high dose of induction agent (Sackeim *et al*, 1991). Other, metabolic, causes were given in Chapter 14. Psychotropic drugs can have important effects on the seizure threshold and the manifestation of cerebral seizure activity (examples are given in Chapter 12). These factors may be important too when the ECT practitioner is faced with a patient with an unusually high initial seizure threshold (see above). It would be good practice to consult with the referring clinical team and anaesthetist to discuss which, if any, of these factors may be modified to ease seizure induction at the next treatment session.

Recommendations

- If the necessary cerebral seizure activity has not been induced, then the patient should be restimulated with a higher electrical dose while still unconscious.
- The extent to which the dose is increased will depend upon whether the ECT practitioner wishes to establish the new, higher seizure threshold, or whether the restimulation is given to maximise the rate of clinical improvement.
- The occurrence of a missed seizure should prompt a review of ECT and anaesthetic technique as well as concomitant psychotropic drug treatment, to identify any factors that may be modified to ease the induction of cerebral seizure activity at the next treatment session.

References

Abrams, R. (2002) *Electroconvulsive Therapy* (4th edn). Oxford: Oxford University Press.

Boylan, L. S., Haskett, R. F., Mulsant, B. H., *et al* (2000) Determinants of seizure threshold in ECT, benzodiazepine use, anaesthetic dosage, and other factors. *Journal of ECT*, **16**, 3–18.

Chung, K. F. & Wong, S. P. (2001) Initial seizure threshold of bilateral electroconvulsive therapy in Chinese. *Journal of ECT*, **17**, 254–258.

Lock, T. (1995) Stimulus dosing. In *The ECT Handbook* (ed. C. P. Freeman), pp. 72–87. London: Royal College of Psychiatrists.

McCall, W. V., Reboussin, D. M., Weiner, R. D., *et al* (2000) Titrated moderately supra-threshold vs fixed high-dose right unilateral electroconvulsive therapy. *Archives of General Psychiatry*, **57**, 438–444.

McCall, W. V., Dunn, A., Rosenquist, P. B., *et al* (2002) Markedly supra-threshold right unilateral ECT versus minimally supra-threshold bilateral ECT: antidepressant and memory affects. *Journal of ECT*, **18**, 126–129.

Robin, A. & De Tissera, S. (1982) A double-blind controlled comparison of the therapeutic effects of low and high energy electroconvulsive therapies. *British Journal of Psychiatry*, **141**, 357–366.

Rose, D., Wykes, T., Leese, M., *et al* (2003) Patients' perspectives on electroconvulsive therapy: systematic review. *British Medical Journal*, **326**, 1363–1365.

Sackeim, H. A., Portnoy, S., Neeley, P., *et al* (1986) Cognitive consequences of low-dosage electroconvulsive therapy. *Annals of the New York Academy of Sciences*, **462**, 326–340.

Sackeim, H. A., Devanand, D. P. & Prudic, J. (1991) Stimulus intensity, seizure threshold and seizure duration: impact on the efficacy and safety of electroconvulsive therapy. *Psychiatric Clinics of North America*, **14**, 803–844.

Sackeim, H. A., Prudic, J., Devanand, D. P., *et al* (1993) Effects of stimulus intensity and electrode placement on the efficacy and cognitive effects of electroconvulsive therapy. *New England Journal of Medicine*, **328**, 839–846.

Sackeim, H. A., Prudic, J., Devanand, D. P., *et al* (2000) A prospective, randomised, double-blind comparison of bilateral and right unilateral electroconvulsive therapy at different stimulus intensities. *Archives of General Psychiatry*, **57**, 425–434.

Scott, A. I. F. & Boddy, H. (2000) The effect of repeated bilateral electroconvulsive therapy on seizure threshold. *Journal of ECT*, **16**, 244–251.

Scott, A. I. F. & Dykes, S. (1999) Initial seizure threshold in the clinical practice of bilateral electroconvulsive therapy in Edinburgh, Scotland. *Journal of ECT*, **15**, 118–124.

Scott, A. I. F., Douglas, R. H. B., Whitfield, A., *et al* (1990) Time course of cerebral magnetic resonance changes after electroconvulsive therapy. *British Journal of Psychiatry*, **156**, 551–553.

Sobin, C., Sackeim, H. A., Prudic, J., *et al* (1995) Predictors of retrograde amnesia following ECT. *American Journal of Psychiatry*, **152**, 995–1001.

UK ECT Review Group (2003) Efficacy and safety of electro-convulsive therapy in depressive disorders: a systematic review and meta-analysis. *Lancet*, **361**, 799–808.

Weiner, R. D., Rogers, H. J., Davidson, J. R. T., *et al* (1986) Effects of stimulus parameters on cognitive side effects. *Annals of the New York Academy of Sciences*, **462**, 315–325.

CHAPTER 17

Monitoring seizure activity

Andrew M. Whitehouse and Allan I. F. Scott

The clinical efficacy of ECT depends on the induction of generalised cerebral seizure activity. The typical seizure is characterised on the electroencephalogram (EEG) by widespread high-frequency spike waves ('polyspike activity') followed by slower spike and wave complexes, typically around 3 cycles per second, or Hertz (Hz). The typical generalised cerebral seizure is followed by a phase of relative or complete suppression of electrical activity ('postictal suppression'). These EEG features are illustrated in Figure 17.1, and discussed in more detail by Weiner *et al* (1991).

The hallmark of generalised cerebral seizure activity is the tonic–clonic, or grand mal, convulsion; after an initial tonic contraction of the muscles, there is a longer, clonic phase of rhythmic alternating contraction and relaxation of the muscles of the limbs on both sides of the body. There may be a delay of a few seconds after the end of electrical stimulation before any convulsion is seen, and this is known as the latent phase.

Several caveats are required. The first aim of anaesthesia for ECT is to produce unconsciousness; intravenous induction agents reduce convulsive activity (Weiner *et al*, 1991). The next aim of anaesthesia is to relax (and sometimes completely to paralyse) voluntary muscles, with the aim of reducing convulsive activity to minimise the risk of physical harm to the patient. Many patients will also be prescribed psychotropic drugs with anticonvulsant properties that alter the induction and manifestation of cerebral seizure activity. Each of these factors promotes a potential dissociation between generalised cerebral seizure activity and visible convulsive activity. Liston *et al* (1988) reviewed ten studies conducted between 1982 and 1987 that reported the ratio of the length of the convulsion to the length of cerebral seizure activity measured by EEG; there was substantial variation in this ratio among the studies, which could not be explained; on average, the length of the convulsion was approximately 70% the length of cerebral seizure activity measured by EEG.

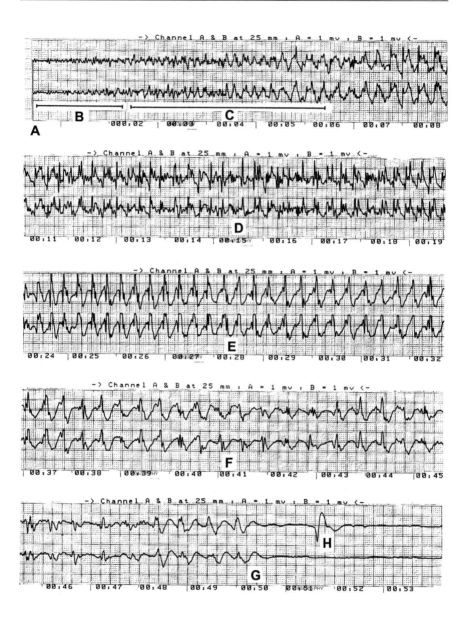

Figure 17.1 EEG features of the necessary generalised cerebral seizure activity. Compare left (top) and right (bottom) hemisphere tracings to confirm generalisation. A: End of electrical stimulation. B: Latent phase – no visible convulsion, only low-amplitude, high-frequency 'polyspike activity' EEG pattern. C: Increasing amplitude of EEG polyspike and gradual slowing of frequency. D: Start of clonic phase of convulsion. E: Classic 3 Hz 'spike and wave' activity. F: Gradual loss of spike and wave pattern. G: End-point, after which EEG tracing has lower amplitude and frequency than at baseline ('postictal suppression'). H: Movement artefact from anaesthetist reapplying face mask.

Seizure duration and clinical efficacy

The length in time of the cerebral seizure activity or the tonic–clonic convulsion is not related to clinical efficacy (Sackeim *et al*, 1991; Weiner *et al*, 1991). The previous edition of the present book acknowledged this, but suggested a clinical guideline, and explicitly not as a firm recommendation, that the treating psychiatrist should question whether or not generalised cerebral seizure activity had occurred if at the first treatment the convulsion lasted less than 15 seconds or the EEG recording showed seizure activity lasting less than 25 seconds (Scott & Lock, 1995). The risk was that such brief convulsive or seizure activity might be the result of a focal or partial seizure, and therefore be of questionable therapeutic efficacy. It was noted none the less that there were patients who recovered with ECT and yet displayed only short tonic–clonic convulsions. This may be more likely in elderly patients (see Chapter 8).

This clinical guideline is no longer valid or relevant. It was suggested at a time when methohexitone was the anaesthetic induction agent of choice. This is no longer commercially available in the UK, and most ECT clinics now use propofol (see Chapter 14), which reduces seizure duration substantially when compared with methohexitone. The aim of ECT is to induce the quality of cerebral seizure activity described at the beginning of this chapter or, in the absence of EEG monitoring, the type of convulsion described above; the quality of the desired activity cannot simply be related to its length in time alone.

Recommendations

- The aim of ECT is to induce the type of generalised cerebral seizure activity described above.
- In the absence of EEG monitoring, or where technical problems mean such monitoring is unreadable, then the aim is to induce tonic–clonic or grand mal convulsive activity on both sides of the body as described above.

Methods of monitoring

Timing of convulsion

It is recommended here that the convulsion be timed from the end of electrical stimulation to the end of generalised, that is, bilateral, clonic activity. If there is a significant discrepancy between the end of generalised clonic activity and the end of clonic activity in one limb, then it would be prudent to record both times. Convulsive activity of the muscles of the face can be seen with focal cerebral seizure activity, and therefore should not be counted if it occurs on its own.

161

If there is no relationship between the length of the convulsion and the clinical efficacy of ECT, then the rationale for the recommendation that the convulsion is timed must be spelled out. It is necessary to remind the reader that unsupervised doctors in training have been observed to take no heed of whether or not a convulsion has been induced (Pippard, 1992). This was one reason for the occurrence of so-called missed seizures; other possible causes are discussed in Chapters 14 and 16. Timing the convulsion at least ensures that the treating doctor heeds whether or not the aim of ECT has been achieved. A brief convulsion ought to prompt the ECT practitioner to ensure that the necessary quality of seizure activity has indeed been induced.

There is another reason to continue to monitor by inspection of the convulsion and this is that it would be incautious to rely on EEG monitoring alone. This method is vulnerable to a number of technical problems: for example, the EEG tracing may be unreadable because it is swamped by artefact, connecting cables may become disconnected, or the machine may unexpectedly run out of paper.

Cuff technique

This is a simple technique that minimises the influence of muscle relaxant on the assessment of convulsive activity. It involves isolating one forearm or leg by inflating a blood pressure cuff to above systolic pressure as the patient is drifting off to sleep, but before the muscle relaxant is administered. If the pressure in the cuff remains above systolic blood pressure, then it isolates the distal part of the limb from the circulating muscle relaxant, allowing unmodified convulsive activity to be observed. It is particularly important to maintain the pressure in the cuff well above systolic pressure seen during seizure activity because if circulating muscle relaxant leaks into the distal part of the limb, it might well be concentrated there, as venous return is occluded. The length of time the cuff is kept inflated is kept to a minimum by deflating it as soon as the convulsion has ended. When unilateral ECT is given, it is suggested the cuff be applied to one of the ipsilateral limbs to ensure that a bilateral convulsion occurs.

This technique is not widely used. This is partly the result of a study that found no difference between the length of the convulsion in cuffed and uncuffed limbs in one English ECT clinic (Wise et al, 2000). While the routine use of the cuff technique cannot be recommended for routine use, it may still be helpful in the management of two clinical scenarios. The first is where only brief convulsive activity has been seen at the outset of the course of treatment, and where EEG monitoring is not available. A substantial proportion of patients who display brief convulsive activity will experience typical generalised cerebral seizure activity, and will therefore not require restimulation or increased electrical dose at the next treatment (Scott *et al*, 1989). The second scenario is where an unusually large dose of muscle relaxant is administered with the aim of total muscle paralysis, for example in a patient who has recently sustained a fracture of a long bone.

EEG monitoring

The previous edition of the handbook noted that EEG monitoring was the most direct available means of measuring seizure activity in the brain itself. A number of major disadvantages of the technique were also listed, for example, that few practitioners in the UK had any experience of the technique, the much higher financial cost of ECT machines with an EEG monitoring facility, and that ECT staff would require extra training and supervision to use it effectively. It was not recommended for routine use, but it was acknowledged that it was underused in the UK and would be of value in particular clinical situations. Two of these were the scenarios described above, that is, where it was desirable to paralyse the patient completely, and in the assessment of brief convulsive activity at the outset of a course of treatment. Another clinical situation was in the detection of prolonged seizures, which might lead to markedly increased cognitive adverse effects without any commensurate therapeutic benefit. This needs more attention now that minimising cognitive adverse effects attributable to ECT has become one of the priorities for contemporary ECT practice.

Prolonged seizures

If seizures are not terminated within 3–5 minutes, then there is a risk of increased confusion and memory impairment. The previous edition of this handbook suggested as a guideline, not as an evidence-based recommendation, that a prolonged seizure was one that lasted 2 minutes or more. The American Psychiatric Association (2001) subsequently suggested a guideline where 3 minutes was used to define a prolonged seizure. There is not a consensus about the definition of a prolonged seizure, but there is agreement that once identified these should be terminated immediately, either by a further dose of induction agent or the intravenous administration of a suitable benzodiazepine drug.

A recent, and challenging, report from India found that 16% of patients experienced prolonged cerebral seizure activity at the first administration of ECT, and in about one-third of cases this was detectable only by EEG monitoring – the convulsion itself was not prolonged (Mayur *et al*, 1999). This study defined prolonged cerebral seizure activity as suggested in the previous edition. These findings, which included the highest prevalence of prolonged cerebral seizure activity ever reported, have been debated. A much lower prevalence was subsequently reported from two Scottish centres that had experimented with EEG monitoring (Scott & McCreadie, 1999); it was suggested special features of the Indian sample might explain this high prevalence, including the large proportion of young people. Abrams (2002) later commented that the high prevalence did not accord with his own clinical experience, and suggested that prolonged cerebral seizure activity was usually seen only where there was some unusual aspect of the patient or the treatment, for example coexisting brain disease. Nevertheless, this study raised two concerns: first, that the prevalence of prolonged cerebral seizure activity may be higher than appreciated, and second, that such prolonged seizures may not be detected if seizure monitoring relies only on the timing of the visible convulsion. Certainly there have been isolated case reports of non-convulsive prolonged cerebral seizure activity or status epilepticus that has been detected only because of simultaneous EEG monitoring (see Scott & Riddle, 1989; Abrams 2002). The risk of prolonged cerebral seizure activity is highest at the first treatment in a course (Sackeim *et al*, 1991; Abrams, 2002).

This topic clearly merits further research, but the Special Committee has decided that the potential risk of undetected prolonged cerebral seizure activity is such that new recommendations must be made before further research findings become available. The major advantage of EEG monitoring is that it is the most direct method for confirming that cerebral seizure activity has ceased. The Committee has therefore decided to recommend that EEG monitoring is provided in all ECT clinics. It is anticipated that it may be a challenge for some clinics where extra training has to be undertaken, or where clinic staff already trained in EEG monitoring do not have adequate dedicated sessional time for ECT duties. For these reasons, the Committee has decided to give warning that this will not be a requirement until 1 January 2006, and acknowledges that it may not be practicable for all clinics to undertake EEG monitoring routinely at all treatments in a course. In the first instance, it may be a reasonable compromise to recommend only that EEG monitoring is available at least at the point in the course of treatment when the risk of prolonged cerebral seizure activity is highest, that is, at the first treatment. This will provide more reliable detection of this potential adverse effect, and also help identify patients in whom there is a marked discrepancy between cerebral seizure activity measured by EEG and the visible convulsion. Patients who experience unusually long cerebral seizure activity at the first treatment, say, seizure activity lasting 1 minute or more, and patients who display an unusually low ratio of convulsive activity to cerebral seizure activity will also require EEG monitoring at least at the second treatment as well.

The necessary cerebral seizure activity is by definition synchronous neuronal activity that is generalised, that is, occurs in both cerebral hemispheres; single-channel EEG recording cannot distinguish focal from generalised cerebral seizure activity. It is also harder to distinguish artefacts from true cerebral seizure activity on a single-channel tracing; for these reasons, single-channel EEG recording is not recommended, and at least one channel from each side of the head is required.

Manufacturers of ECT machines can supply self-adhesive, pre-gelled, disposable EEG electrodes. Most ECT practitioners prefer to position these away from the hairy scalp and far apart, to maximise the amplitude of the EEG tracing, that is, just above the middle of the eyebrow on the forehead and on the skin over the ipsilateral mastoid process, the so-called prefrontal–mastoid positioning.

Recommendations

- Prolonged cerebral seizure activity is a recognised adverse effect of ECT; it increases the risk of adverse cognitive effects, without any commensurate increase in clinical efficacy. These are treatable, if detected.
- The most direct method to detect prolonged cerebral seizure activity is EEG monitoring. It is for this reason that the Special Committee on ECT has decided to recommend that EEG monitoring must be available in all ECT clinics from 1 January 2006.
- Single-channel EEG monitoring is not recommended: at least one channel from each side of the head is required.
- It is appreciated that it may be a challenge for all clinics to monitor all treatments in a course by EEG monitoring. The risk of prolonged cerebral seizure activity is greatest at the first treatment, and as an interim development it may be sufficient that EEG monitoring is always carried out at the first treatment only.
- EEG monitoring is prudent beyond the first treatment for patients with unusually long cerebral seizure activity at the first treatment or where the ratio of the length of convulsive activity to cerebral seizure activity is unusually low.
- Revised recommendations about the methods of monitoring cerebral seizure activity are summarised in Table 17.1.

Assessment of seizure adequacy by EEG

It was noted in Chapter 16 that the seizure threshold may, but will not inevitably, rise over a course of treatment, and if this happened, then the electrical dose should rise *pari passu* to maintain the dosing strategy. It was also noted that, in the absence of obvious evidence such as a missed seizure, any change in the length of the convulsions was only

Table 17.1 Methods of monitoring seizure activity

Method	Advantages	Disadvantages	Recommendations
Timing of convulsion	Simple, cheap and ensures that the treating psychiatrist confirms that a tonic–clonic convulsion has been induced	Seizure activity may be confused with muscle contraction during stimulation. It is heavily influenced by muscle relaxant, and may be abolished by the same. It under-estimates cerebral seizure activity	Minimum requirement in all ECT suites
Cuff technique	Cheap and unaffected by muscle relaxant	Cuff pressure needs continual maintenance. It may be left inflated after ECT. There is a risk of trauma in frail patients and there is a risk of clotting in patients with sickle-cell disease. It underestimates cerebral seizure activity	It is useful in the assessment of brief convulsions. It is valuable when total paralysis is desirable and when EEG monitoring is unavailable
EEG	Most direct assessment of cerebral seizure activity. It can detect both focal and prolonged seizures. Research, e.g. prevalence of prolonged seizures	Cost (doubles the cost of an ECT machine, plus there is the cost of consumables such as disposable electrodes and graph paper). It requires training and supervision. A single-channel reading cannot detect focal seizures, and is prone to artefacts	To be available in all clinics from 1 January 2006. At least one channel from each side of the head is needed. Where lack of human resources makes routine monitoring impracticable, the minimum requirement is that it is carried out at the first treatment

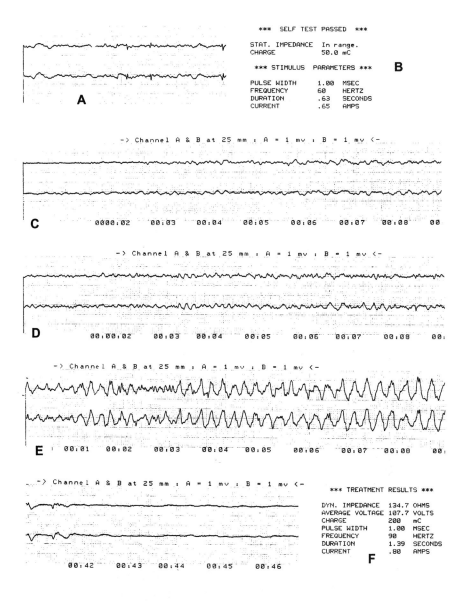

Figure 17.2 EEG tracing from Mecta SR2 ECT machine. A: Baseline α rhythm, 8–12 Hz. B: Self-test result at setting for first stimulation (50 mC). C: First stimulation is below the seizure threshold, and there is no visible convulsion and no significant alteration in the EEG pattern. D: Patient is restimulated with higher dose (75 mC); there is still no visible convulsion and still no significant alteration in EEG pattern. E: Patient restimulated with a substantially higher dose (200 mC), which results in a generalised tonic–clonic convulsion lasting 22 seconds, and necessary generalised cerebral seizure activity lasting 41 seconds. F: Automatic print-out at end of the treatment session.

modestly correlated with any rise in the seizure threshold; clinical monitoring remained the best guide to what, if any, change in electrical dose was required. There has been much research interest in the potential of EEG monitoring to contribute to the assessment of seizure adequacy; unfortunately, this is a potential yet to be fulfilled. Once the necessary cerebral seizure activity has been induced and recorded by EEG, it is not yet possible for the ECT practitioner to examine an individual EEG tracing and make accurate predictions about the clinical outcome after a course of treatment (see Nobler *et al*, 2000). Nevertheless, the availability of EEG monitoring may contribute to decisions about the need to increase the electrical dose over a course of treatment. If high-amplitude synchronous typical cerebral seizure activity and typical postictal suppression appear on EEG early in the course of treatment, but progressively the EEG tracings show less clear-cut or fewer typical features, then this may suggest that the electrical dose is gradually becoming less supra-threshold as the seizure threshold rises. Progressive EEG changes must, however, be assessed in the context of the necessary clinical monitoring; the ECT practitioner is treating the patient, not the EEG tracing. Figure 17.2 contrasts the EEG tracings from doses below and above the initial seizure threshold.

References

Abrams, R. (2002) *Electroconvulsive Therapy* (4th edn). Oxford: Oxford University Press.

American Psychiatric Association (2001) *The Practice of Electroconvulsive ECT: Recommendations for Treatment, Training and Privileging* (2nd edn). Washington, DC: APA.

Liston, E. H., Guze, B. H., Baxter, L. R., *et al* (1988) Motor versus EEG seizure duration in ECT. *Biological Psychiatry*, **24**, 94–96.

Mayur, P. M., Gangadhar, B. N., Janakiramaiah, N., *et al* (1999) Motor seizure monitoring during electroconvulsive therapy. *British Journal of Psychiatry*, **174**, 270–272.

Nobler, M. S., Luber, B., Moeller, J. R., *et al* (2000) Quantitative EEG during seizures induced by electroconvulsive therapy: relations to treatment modality and clinical features. I. Global analyses. *Journal of ECT*, **16**, 211–228.

Pippard, J. (1992) Audit of electroconvulsive treatment in two national health service regions. *British Journal of Psychiatry*, **160**, 621–637.

Sackeim, H. A., Devanand, D. P. & Prudic, J. (1991) Stimulus intensity, seizure threshold, and seizure duration: impact on the efficacy and safety of electroconvulsive therapy. *Psychiatric Clinics of North America*, **14**, 843–844.

Scott, A. I. & Lock, T. (1995) Monitoring seizure activity. In *The ECT Handbook* (1st edn) (ed. C. P. Freeman), pp. 62–66. London: Royal College of Psychiatrists.

Scott, A. I. & McCreadie, R. G. (1999) Prolonged seizures detectable by electroencephalogram in electroconvulsive therapy (letter). *British Journal of Psychiatry*, **175**, 91–92.

Scott, A. I. & Riddle, W. (1989) Status epilepticus after electroconvulsive therapy. *British Journal of Psychiatry*, **155**, 119–121.

Scott, A. I., Shering, P. A. & Dykes, S. (1989) Would monitoring by electroencephalogram improve the practice of electroconvulsive therapy? *British Journal of Psychiatry*, **154**, 853–857.

Weiner, R. D., Coffey, C. E. & Krystal, A. D. (1991) The monitoring and management of electrically induced seizures. *Psychiatric Clinics of North America*, **14**, 845–870.

Wise, M. E. J., Mackie, F., Zamar, A. C., *et al* (2000) Investigation of the 'cuff' method for assessing seizure duration in electroconvulsive therapy. *Psychiatric Bulletin*, **24**, 301.

CHAPTER 18

Adverse effects of ECT

Susan M. Benbow

Assessment before ECT

The adverse effects of ECT are a major concern for people treated with ECT, their families and the public. During the assessment process, before the person consents to treatment, the risk–benefit balance for a particular person will be considered and discussed. If there are reasons why this person might be at greater risk of particular adverse effects, ways in which the risk might be minimised should be considered. For example, people with a concurrent dementia may be at increased risk of developing cognitive adverse effects during ECT (Griesemer *et al*, 1997; Krystal & Coffey, 1997) and for this reason unilateral ECT may be preferred to bilateral ECT in these circumstances. Similarly, people with existing cardiac disease may be at risk of adverse cardiac events during treatment and therefore may be treated in a cardiac care unit with specialist staff to hand (see Chapter 7).

Informed consent

As far as possible, patients and their families should be involved in discussions about the treatment, its likely adverse effects, its possible benefits, any alternative treatments and the risks (if any) of not having the treatment. The use of written as well as verbal information is good practice.

Mortality rate

Electroconvulsive therapy is a low-risk procedure with a mortality rate similar to that of anaesthesia for minor surgical procedures, despite its frequent use in elderly people and those with major medical problems (Sackeim, 1998; Weiner *et al*, 2000). The American Psychiatric Association (2001) stated that a reasonable current estimate of the ECT-related mortality rate is 1 per 10 000 patients or 1 per 80 000 treatments. This must be set in the context of any risks involved in not having ECT. For some people, morbidity and mortality rates with ECT are believed to be lower than with some antidepressive drug treatments (Sackeim, 1998).

Cardiovascular and pulmonary complications are the most likely causes of death and serious morbidity. Patients identified as being at high risk should be closely monitored and treated in an environment that will allow rapid intervention should complications occur (see Chapter 7).

Prolonged seizures

Prolonged seizures and status epilepticus are more likely in people on medication that lowers their seizure threshold, such as theophylline (Abrams, 2002), or with pre-existing medical conditions that lower their seizure threshold, such as electrolyte imbalance (Finlayson et al, 1989). Non-convulsive status epilepticus following ECT may be difficult to diagnose; EEG monitoring will indicate whether or not seizure activity has ceased (Weiner & Krystal, 1993).

Cognitive adverse effects

Cognitive adverse effects are the main concern for many people, and orientation and memory should be assessed before and at intervals throughout the course of treatment. Recent reviews of the literature on cognitive adverse effects have been cited by the UK ECT Review Group (see Chapter 2) and the American Psychiatric Association (2001). ECT can affect memory for events that occurred before ECT (retrograde amnesia) and events that take place after ECT (anterograde amnesia). Recent evidence has suggested that retrograde amnesia is greater for impersonal than for personal memory (Lisanby et al, 2000). The ability to learn new information and non-memory cognitive functions (intelligence, judgement, abstraction, etc.) are not affected. Severe depressive illness, particularly in older adults, can affect memory, and tests of memory carried out before and after ECT may show improvement, presumably because the memory deficits associated with depression have improved in response to treatment (Coleman et al, 1996).

Weiner (2000) recently summarised our knowledge regarding the retrograde amnesia that can occur with ECT and noted that:

- ECT produces deficits in both autobiographical and impersonal memory domains
- these losses improve substantially after completion of an ECT course, but residual difficulties persist in some patients

- the severity and persistence of retrograde amnesia is greater with bilateral electrode placement than with unilateral non-dominant electrode placement, and with sine-wave stimuli than with pulse stimuli
- the extent of the retrograde amnesia is not significantly correlated with the degree of therapeutic improvement
- the relationship between objective measures and self-reports of retrograde amnesia is complex, with the latter tending to be more highly correlated with therapeutic outcome than with objective test results.

Objective memory impairment (i.e. impairment that can be demonstrated on objective tests) occurring during a course of ECT is generally reversible, but a small proportion of people complain of persisting memory difficulty after treatment and may have persisting loss of memory for events during a period before, during and after ECT (Lisanby et al, 2000; Sackeim et al, 2000).

Fink (1999) argues that depressive illness and psychotropic drugs affect memory, but that, when ECT is used, any detrimental effects are blamed solely on the ECT, which then bears the full burden of public fear of the cognitive effects related to psychiatric treatment.

The most marked cognitive adverse effects occur immediately postictally, when people experience a variable period of disorientation, associated with impaired attention, memory and praxis (Sackeim, 1986). These effects resolve over time and are normally short-lived.

The ECT technique affects the type and severity of adverse cognitive effects. Stimulus waveform, stimulus intensity, electrode placement, inter-ECT interval, concomitant drug treatment and anaesthetic medication all affect the severity of adverse cognitive effects. Increased cognitive adverse effects are associated with sine-wave treatment, bilateral electrode placement, high stimulus intensity in relation to individual seizure threshold, short inter-ECT interval, certain concomitant drug treatments (including lithium) and high doses of anaesthetic medication. It follows that actions that might be expected to decrease cognitive adverse effects include: changing to brief-pulse stimulation, using unilateral electrode placement, lowering stimulus intensity in relation to individual seizure threshold, lengthening the inter-ECT interval, decreasing or stopping concomitant drug treatments, and reducing anaesthetic drug doses (where possible).

Acute confusional states may develop between treatments, particularly in people taking concurrent psychotropic drugs, or those with pre-existing cognitive impairment or neurological conditions. If this occurs, modifications to treatment technique may lessen the confusion. Rarely a person will develop postictal delirium (Devanand et al, 1989), which can manifest as restlessness, aggression or agitation in the early stages of recovery. This will respond to treatment with benzodiazepines.

Other adverse effects

After treatment, people may suffer from headaches, muscular aches, drowsiness, weakness, nausea and anorexia. These are usually only mild and respond to symptomatic treatments. People who commonly experience post-ECT headaches may benefit from prophylactic treatment immediately after ECT (e.g. aspirin or a non-steroidal anti-inflammatory drug).

Adverse psychological reactions to ECT are rare, but may involve the person developing an intense fear of treatment (Fox, 1993). Support and information are critical in preventing and managing this side-effect of treatment.

Regular review during the course of treatment

Regular review is necessary during the course of treatment to detect the possible adverse effects listed above. If detected, this should prompt consideration of whether these could be avoided, minimised or treated. Staff of the ECT clinic, in conjunction with ward staff caring for those people being treated with ECT, may wish to develop and use standardised assessments of possible treatment-emergent adverse effects.

Recommendations

- During pre-ECT assessment, ways of minimising potential adverse effects should be considered, particularly for those people who are deemed at high risk of adverse effects during treatment.
- During the consent process, patients should be informed of the likely adverse effects related to treatment within the context of considering the risks and benefits of treatment.
- Doctors prescribing or administering ECT should be aware of particular possible adverse effects of treatment.
- All ECT clinics should have a protocol for the management of prolonged seizures (see Chapter 17).
- Orientation and memory should be assessed before and after the first ECT, and re-assessed at intervals throughout treatment course.
- People receiving ECT should be regularly reviewed during the course of treatment, when attention should be given to possible treatment-emergent adverse effects. Ways of preventing, minimising and treating adverse effects should be considered.

References

Abrams, R. (2002) *Electroconvulsive Therapy* (4th edn). New York: Oxford University Press.

American Psychiatric Association (2001) Adverse effects. In *The Practice of Electro-convulsive Therapy: Recommendations for Treatment, Training and Privileging* (2nd edn), pp. 59–76. Washington, DC: APA.

Coleman, E. A., Sackeim, H. A., Prudic, J., *et al* (1996) Subjective memory complaints before and after electroconvulsive therapy. *Biological Psychiatry*, **39**, 346–356.

Devanand, D. P., Briscoe, K. M. & Sackeim, H. A. (1989) Clinical features and predictors of post-ictal excitement. *Convulsive Therapy*, **5**, 140–146.

Fink, M. (1999) *Electroshock: Restoring the Mind.* Oxford: Oxford University Press.

Finlayson, A. J., Vieweg, W. V., Wiley, W. D., *et al* (1989) Hyponatraemic seizure following ECT. *Canadian Journal of Psychiatry*, **34**, 463–464.

Fox, H. A. (1993) Patients' fear of and objection to electroconvulsive therapy. *Hospital and Community Psychiatry*, **44**, 357–360.

Griesemer, D. A., Kellner, C. H., Beale, M. D., *et al* (1997) Electroconvulsive therapy for treatment of intractable seizures: initial findings in two children. *Neurology*, **49**, 1389–1392.

Krystal, A. D. & Coffey, C. E. (1997) Neuropsychiatric considerations in the use of electroconvulsive therapy. *Journal of Neuropsychiatry and Clinical Neurosciences*, **9**, 283–292.

Lisanby, S. H., Maddox, J. H., Prudic, J., *et al* (2000) The effects of electroconvulsive therapy on memory of autobiographical and public events. *Archives of General Psychiatry*, **57**, 581–590.

Sackeim, H. A. (1986) Acute cognitive side-effects of ECT. *Psychopharmacology Bulletin*, **22**, 482–484.

Sackeim, H. A. (1998) The use of electroconvulsive therapy in late-life depression. In *Geriatric Psychopharmacology* (3rd edn) (ed. C. Salzman), pp. 262–309. Baltimore, MD: Williams & Wilkins.

Sackeim, H. A., Prudic, J., Devanand, D. P., *et al* (2000) A prospective, randomized, double-blind comparison of bilateral and right unilateral electroconvulsive therapy at different stimulus intensities. *Archives of General Psychiatry*, **57**, 425–434.

Weiner, R. D. (2000) Retrograde amnesia with electroconvulsive therapy: characteristics and implications. *Archives of General Psychiatry*, **57**, 591–592.

Weiner, R. D. & Krystal, A. D. (1993) EEG monitoring of ECT seizures. In *The Clinical Science of Electroconvulsive Therapy* (ed. C. E. Coffey), pp. 93–109. Washington, DC: APA.

Weiner, R. D., Coffey, C. E. & Krystal, A. D. (2000) Electroconvulsive therapy in the medical and neurologic patient. In *Psychiatric Care of the Medical Patient* (2nd edn) (eds A. Stoudemire, B. S. Fogel & D. Greenberg), pp. 419–428. New York: Oxford University Press.

CHAPTER 19

Training, supervision and professional development

Richard Duffett, Grace M. Fergusson and Martin Stevens

For each ECT clinic there needs to be a consultant who takes a lead in the development of the service. The role of this consultant can be considered in five areas:

- development of treatment protocols
- training and supervision of clinical staff
- advice and liaison with other professionals
- audit and quality assurance
- continuing professional development.

Even for a small ECT clinic, fulfilling adequately these roles is likely to demand a significant time commitment and for that reason the Royal College of Psychiatrists (1999) stated that the consultant psychiatrist has to have designated time in the job plan to fulfil these roles. Day-to-day responsibility may be delegated to other senior staff (e.g. a specialist registrar as part of their training), or a non-training-grade experienced psychiatrist, but a designated consultant does need to retain overall responsibility.

Development of treatment protocols

The consultant responsible for an ECT clinic is the key individual in developing a written treatment protocol that details how patients should be stimulated (e.g. whether unilateral or bilateral electrode placement should be used in what sort of cases) and what procedures should be followed in the event of missed or prolonged seizures. Reviews of the treatment protocol will be required in light of local audit findings, new guidance from the College or in response to new research. In addition, the designated consultant will need to develop protocols for the prescription of ECT by his or her peers (ensuring treatments are prescribed individually or in pairs); protocols should ensure that adequate anaesthetic assessment occurs and information about a patient's clinical response is communicated to the doctor administering ECT. The consultant psychiatrist also has a role to play in ensuring that anaesthetic protocols are adapted to meet the needs of patients receiving ECT and that nursing protocols are in line with recommendations in the present book, for example. In conclusion, the ECT consultant must share in the clinical responsibility for each patient undergoing treatment.

Training and supervision

The consultant responsible for the ECT clinic must ensure that doctors involved in administering ECT have been suitably trained and are subject to ongoing supervision. This includes the assessment and training of doctors new to the ECT roster, even if they have received training elsewhere. Individuals vary in the amount of time they need to become competent in the delivery of ECT and the responsible consultant needs to satisfy himself or herself that any doctor administering ECT without direct supervision has reached a satisfactory level of knowledge. The following would be integral to the training of those involved in administering ECT:

- an introduction to the theoretical basis of effective treatment with ECT
- familiarity with the local ECT protocol and clinic layout
- observation of the administration of ECT before they administer it themselves
- directly supervised administration of ECT at least three times before unsupervised administration is undertaken
- supervision directly or through the examination of treatment charts at least once a week while they are administering ECT
- the opportunity to appraise papers on ECT, most likely as part of the regular journal club.

Advice and liaison with other professionals

Liaison with others involved with ECT is essential in drawing up a protocol for the clinic. Once this is done it is likely that ongoing meetings will be required to ensure the smooth operation of the clinic. These meetings may require management input when issues around capital expenditure or staffing arise.

Audit and quality assurance

Standards for the administration of ECT have been criticised by successive audits conducted by the Royal College of Psychiatrists

(Duffett & Lelliott, 1998). As ECT is administered to very ill patients and it is a procedure involving the risks of a general anaesthetic, it is important to ensure that it is given effectively. Audits examining one or more aspects of the clinic's operation may lead to modifications of treatment protocols. It should not be assumed just by having a protocol that it will be followed. Methods of ensuring that treatment is administered to a high standard include direct observation of doctors administering ECT (which may reveal poor technique, such as the removal of live electrodes). The review of treatment charts, particularly when missed seizures have occurred, may also highlight the need for further training.

In May 2003, to coincide with the publication of the guidance from the National Institute for Clinical Excellence (see Chapter 1), the Royal College of Psychiatrists announced that it was to launch a new ECT Accreditation Service (ECTAS), which was to be managed by the College Research Unit. The aim was to raise standards in the administration of ECT by a process of self-review and external review involving psychiatrists, nurses, anaesthetists and lay representatives. The first edition of the ECTAS standards for the administration of ECT was published in December 2003 and is available online at the following website: www.rcpsych.ac.uk/cru/ECTAS.htm.

Continuing professional development

Consultants involved with ECT clinics need to ensure their knowledge is updated. There are now local approved theoretical and practical training days in many parts of the country. Guidance has been updated between ECT handbooks in Council Reports (CR73) and articles in the *Psychiatric Bulletin*. It is likely that this practice will continue. ECT training days outlining the basics of ECT have been run since 1992 by the Royal College of Psychiatrists through its Special Committee on ECT. These will now be supplemented by national meetings for experienced ECT practitioners, which will provide a forum for networking and discussion of controversies in treatment. Sessions on ECT have occurred about once every 2 years at annual meetings of the Royal College of Psychiatrists.

References

Duffett, R. & Lelliott, P. (1998) Auditing electroconvulsive therapy. The third cycle. *British Journal of Psychiatry*, **172**, 401–405.

Royal College of Psychiatrists (1999) *Guidelines for Healthcare Commissioners for an ECT Service* (Council Report CR73). London: Royal College of Psychiatrists.

Part IV
The law and consent

CHAPTER 20

The law and consent to treatment[*]

Richard Barnes, Jim A. T. Dyer, Roy J. McClelland
and Allan I. F. Scott

All medical procedures, be they therapeutic or investigative, touch upon the issue of consent – that is, a measure of willingness on the part of the patient to undertake the procedure proposed. In this, ECT is no different to the majority of therapeutic interventions. However, ECT has a particular status both within psychiatry and within the law that makes specific discussion of issues with regard to consent worthwhile.

In 1995 the previous edition of the present work noted that practice and regulations about consent to ECT were broadly similar throughout the UK. Consent to treatment in the Republic of Ireland was considered separately, and this is still reasonable. Scotland now needs to be considered separately too, because of the implementation of the Adults with Incapacity (Scotland) Act 2000 from July 2002 and because the Scottish Parliament's Mental Health (Care and Treatment) (Scotland) Act 2003 is expected to be implemented from April 2005. New legislation to address the rights of people incapacitated by mental disorder is being considered across the other countries of the UK and also in the Republic of Ireland; it is likely there will be either changes to existing legislation or new legislation in the next few years.

England and Wales, and Northern Ireland

Leaving aside exceptions provided for detained patients (see below), it is unlawful and unethical to treat a patient who is capable of understanding and willing to know, without first explaining the nature of any procedure, its purpose and implications, and obtaining that person's agreement. This also applies to patients who choose to remain ignorant of the full details of their diagnosis and treatment, so long as they have the option of receiving this information.

---

[*]This chapter includes some material that was in the previous edition, which was written by Dr John Pippard and Professor Pamela Taylor.

The first stage of obtaining consent must always be an assessment of a patient's capacity to give that consent. The current legal test of capacity holds that an adult has capacity to consent (or refuse consent) to medical treatment if he or she can:

- understand and retain the information relevant to the decision in question
- believe that information
- weigh that information in the balance to arrive at a choice.

When providing that information, the doctor must ensure the individual can:

- understand what the medical treatment is, its purpose and nature, and why it is being proposed
- understand its principal benefits, risks and alternatives
- understand in broad terms what will be the consequences of not receiving the proposed treatment
- retain the information for long enough to make an effective decision
- make a free choice (free from pressure).

Since obtaining consent thus involves an assessment of capacity, it is best done by a senior clinician (i.e. the patient's consultant).

While it is important that patients are able broadly to understand the implications of refusing a treatment, this should not be used as a form of coercion to persuade reluctant patients to accept ECT (e.g. 'If you don't consent, then there's nothing more I will do'). The law is clear that any form of coercion would negate the validity of the consent and is also unethical. Similarly, it is unacceptable under any circumstances to use the threat of enforced treatment under a section of the Mental Health Act to obtain informed consent. As part of the discussion, alternative therapies to ECT should be raised and it should be made clear that a refusal of treatment will not prejudice the further care of that patient.

Consent to a course of ECT is unusual in that written consent is obtained for the course of treatment and not for each treatment session. It is important, therefore, to ensure patients clearly understand that consent can be withheld at any time, despite a consent form having been signed. They should also understand how they might inform staff about a change in consent. The continuation of consent should be verbally checked before each treatment. It is good practice for consent forms to include a fixed number of treatments to which the patient is consenting. This figure can be negotiated with individual patients, although the arbitrary figure of 12 has been suggested as a standard. Further treatment beyond this agreed figure would require another written consent form.

ECT without patient consent

The proportion of patients receiving ECT without giving valid consent is small, but significant. After a patient and the consultant have had discussions regarding ECT, there are four situations in which consent may not have been obtained:

- The patient has the capacity to give consent but chooses not to do so.
- The patient is unable to consent and there is 'necessity' to treat.
- The patient lacks the capacity to consent because of a mental disorder and is not compliant with the proposed treatment.
- The patient lacks the capacity to consent and is compliant with the treatment plan.

The capacitated patient withholding consent

Here the patient can make a decision and decides to say 'no'.

The common law is that a person of full age and sound under-standing may choose to reject medical advice and medical or surgical treatment either partially or in its entirety. A decision to refuse medical treatment by a person capable of making the decision does not have to be sensible, rational or well considered. It would be possible in certain circumstances to use the existing mental health legislation to adminis-ter ECT to a detained patient who is mentally able to give valid informed consent and who refused to consent to ECT. Neither the authors of this chapter nor the Royal College of Psychiatrists' Special Committee on ECT would consider this good practice.

Treatment out of 'necessity'

Here the patient is in a life-threatening situation and cannot consent, for example because unconscious.

The concept of 'necessity' permits doctors to provide treatment without obtaining the patient's consent provided that: there is a need to act when it is not practical to communicate with the assisted person; and also the action taken must be such as a reasonable person would in all the circumstances take acting in the best interests of the assisted person. Hence, not only is a doctor able to give treatment to an incapacitated patient when it is clearly in that patient's best interest, but it is a common law duty to do so. However, this applies only to treatment carried out to ensure improvement or prevent deterioration in health and should be used only before the patient can be in a position to decide for himself or herself. It is essential that if someone now incapacitated is known to have objection to some, or all, of a treatment, that these objections are considered, even in an emergency. It is good practice to obtain a second opinion regarding 'necessity' before proceeding with a treatment.

ECT in the incapacitated non-compliant patient

Here a patient says 'no' but is sufficiently mentally ill to prevent a proper understanding of what is being proposed and why.

For a patient incapacitated by reason of mental disorder it is permissible to administer ECT under the auspices of the appropriate Mental Health Act. In England and Wales, ECT is governed by the provisions of Part IV of the Mental Health Act 1983 (section 58). In Northern Ireland, it is governed by the provisions of Part IV of the Mental Health (Northern Ireland) Order 1986 (article 64). In order for these provisions to be applied, a medical practitioner appointed for the purpose by the Mental Health Act Commission or Mental Health Commission for Northern Ireland should have assessed the detained patient and authorised the plan for treatment. This is recorded on 'form 39' (England and Wales) or 'form 23' (Northern Ireland) and sent to the relevant Commission. It is a requirement that the proposed maximum number of treatment sessions is specified.

When emergency or urgent treatment is required, treatment may be given under section 62 of the Act or article 68 of the Order. Detained patients may be given any treatment, including ECT, which is immediately necessary for one of the following purposes:

- to save the patient's life
- to prevent a serious deterioration (not being irreversible)
- to alleviate serious suffering (not being irreversible or hazardous)
- as the minimum necessary to prevent the patient from behaving violently or being a danger to himself or herself or to others (not being irreversible or hazardous).

It could be argued that ECT is given legitimately under any or all of these provisions for urgent treatment. It has not been stated in statute law that ECT is to be regarded as either irreversible or hazardous. ECT is not a treatment that is intrinsically irreversible, like neurosurgery for mental disorder. The potential hazard of treatment will vary substantially among patients and be estimated by the clinical assessment of the risks of anaesthesia and ECT in the context of the individual patient's general health or coexisting medical conditions. Nevertheless, the present authors would emphasise that these provisions for urgent treatment of detained patients allow the statutory processes of consent to or authorisation of ECT to be bypassed by the practitioner. It is the view of the authors that this should be done only rarely and only in extremis. The authors and the Special Committee would therefore recommend that, in the case of ECT, these provisions for urgent treatment be used solely to save the patient's life.

In England and Wales, the Mental Health Act Commission should be informed as soon as possible that urgent treatment with ECT is proposed, so that a medical practitioner can be appointed by the

Commission. In Northern Ireland, it is a statutory requirement that the responsible medical officer (RMO) immediately notifies the Commission as to the nature of the treatment given to the patient, and which of the four possible indications for urgent treatment applied to the patient.

Medical practitioners appointed by either Commission can usually attend promptly and hopefully repeated use of section 62 or article 68 for an individual patient will not be required; if this were being considered, then it would be essential to reassess whether or not the above conditions for urgent treatment still pertained.

ECT in the incapacitated compliant patient

Here the patient is sufficiently mentally ill to prevent a proper understanding of what is being proposed and why, but does not indicate an unwillingness to accept the treatment.

Until recently, it was customary to consider detention, partly to allow external scrutiny of the proposed treatment and partly to provide a legal template by way of the parts of the Mental Health Acts relating to consent to treatment. At the time of writing, this is still the practice in Northern Ireland, but a change of practice has been suggested in England and Wales. In a recent edition of the *Mental Health Act Manual* (Jones, 1999) it is argued that:

as the provision of medical treatment to a mentally incapable patient is authorised under the common law if the treatment, which can be for a physical or a psychiatric disorder, is considered to be in the patient's best interests, the 'sectioning' of the patient for the purpose of providing 'authority' for medical treatment for his mental disorder to be given, is unnecessary. Such action is almost certainly unlawful because the 'sectioning' of a compliant incapable patient would not be 'warranted' for the purposes of Section 2 and it would not be possible to satisfy the requirements in Section 3 that the treatment 'cannot be provided' unless the patient is detained under that Section. The detention of a compliant mentally incapable informal patient is authorised under the common law doctrine of 'necessity.'

This follows on from the 'Bournewood' judgement, where it was determined that an incapacitated compliant patient need not be detained under the Mental Health Act (*R* v. *Bournewood Community and Mental Health NHS Trust ex parte L*, 1998 All ER 319). It thus follows, so the argument goes, that any treatment of patients in these circumstances could be dealt with under the doctrine of 'necessity'. Most clinicians seem uncomfortable with prescribing ECT in these circumstances, where there is no consent from the patient or second opinion under the Mental Health Act. The legality of ECT in these circumstances has not, at the time of writing, been tested in the courts. If this clinical situation is thought to arise, the following are suggested as best practice:

- Attempts should be made to improve the patient's clinical condition so he or she is able to consent to the treatment proposed.
- If this is not possible, the patient should be seen by the consultant and a formal assessment of his or her capacity and compliance made.
- Capacity should be assessed according to the guidance given above. When assessing compliance, the doctor should consider whether the patient is compliant with other aspects of treatment and if he or she is likely to resist ECT.
- If the patient is incapacitated yet compliant, the prescribing doctor should discuss the findings with appropriate family and carers whenever possible. A second opinion from a consultant colleague should also be sought.
- Once this has been done the doctor should clearly document that the patient is incapacitated yet compliant and arrangements be made with the ECT service to administer one treatment.
- The patient should be reassessed following each treatment with regard to both capacity and compliance.

At subsequent assessment the possible outcomes would be as follows:
- The patients develops the capacity to consent and either:
  - agrees to the treatment, in which case the patient should complete a normal consent form in order to allow treatment to proceed
  - withholds consent to treatment, in which case the decision should then be made either to withhold the ECT or to proceed with assessment for detention under section 2 or 3 before the treatment is given under section 58.
- The patient remains incapacitated and either:
  - indicates a lack of compliance with the treatment in word or deed, in which case assessment for detention under section 3 should be made before treatment is given under section 58, as the patient is no longer incapacitated and compliant
  - remains compliant, in which case, again, this should be clearly documented in the case notes to allow a further treatment to be given.

At all times a dialogue should take place between prescribing doctor, approved social worker, family and patient, to ensure that the number of treatments given under these circumstances is minimised.

ECT for capacitated detained patients

Some patients considered for ECT may already be detained and subject to the provisions of Part IV of the Act or Order. Nevertheless, they are considered able to give valid informed consent to ECT; for example, they may be detained for the treatment of schizophrenia but have subsequently also developed a severe depressive illness. In these circumstances the provisions of section 58 or article 64 still apply, and the capacitated consent will need to be formally recorded on form 38 (England and Wales) or form 23 (Northern Ireland) before treatment can begin. The RMO must complete a certificate that states that the patient is capable of understanding the nature, purpose and likely effects of the treatment. The proposed maximum number of treatment sessions must be specified.

Scotland

The consent of the patient is an important issue in relation to any treatment. Public controversy surrounding ECT gives added emphasis to the need for the treatment to be given according to good practice guidelines (e.g. Clinical Resource and Audit Group, Working Group on Mental Illness, 1997). Both good practice and lawful practice require close attention to the issue of consent.

The Mental Welfare Commission for Scotland has issued guidance on consent issues for ECT coordinators (Mental Welfare Commission for Scotland, 1999) which emphasises that 'no patient should be treated with ECT unless there has been careful consideration of the consent issues and proper and lawful procedures have been followed to obtain consent, or, in the absence of consent, lawful authority to proceed'.

Conditions requiring treatment with ECT, most typically severe depressive illness, may remove or impair the capacity of the patient to give informed consent. The most extreme example might be a depressive stupor. A patient with depression may also have difficulty absorbing information about ECT and coming to a decision, or the psychopathology of depression may lead a patient to welcome ECT as a punishment or something that will hasten death. An agreement given in such circumstances would not constitute valid consent. Despite this, most people currently receiving ECT in Scotland are considered able to give informed consent. The National Audit of ECT in Scotland (Freeman et al, 2000) showed that around 1000 people each year receive ECT and of these over 80% give consent. Recent annual reports of the Mental Welfare Commission for Scotland (e.g. Mental Welfare Commission for Scotland, 2003) show that detained patients subject to Part X of the Mental Health (Scotland) Act 1984 account for around a quarter to a fifth of courses of ECT administered annually, but even in these detained patients about 20% have their consent to treatment indicated on 'form 9'.

Informal (non-detained) patients

Patient capable of consenting

Informal patients capable of consenting to, or refusing, treatment should receive ECT only with their free and informed consent. This is generally taken to mean that the patient understands what the treatment entails and its purpose and likely effects, both beneficial and adverse. Explanations should be given in terms that the patient is able to understand. The patient should also understand what any other treatment options might be and the likely effects of not having the ECT. Capacity and incapacity must be regarded as dynamic concepts which can change over time and are not to be considered 'all or nothing' phenomena. Capacity to manage financial affairs, to take personal welfare decisions, to consent to treatment and so on must all be considered separately and in a situation-specific fashion. A patient may be able to consent to a simple treatment but not to a more complex one. The patient should be advised, if consent is given, that it may later be withdrawn. Consent must be considered in relation to each individual ECT treatment, although separate documentation is not necessary for each treatment.

If the doctor in charge of the patient's treatment is satisfied that real consent can be and has been given, the patient should be asked to sign a standard consent form, and the doctor should also sign. The form provides evidence that consent has been sought but not of the validity of that consent. It is therefore advisable to make a note in the case record of the interview at which consent was obtained. Consent should be for up to a limited and stated number of treatments given, with a stated frequency. The National Audit Team is producing a new consent form that records this. If there is a gap of more than 2 weeks between consent and the start of treatment, fresh consent procedures should be followed and if there is a break of more than 2 weeks in the course of treatments the subsequent treatments should be regarded as a fresh course for which new consent procedures are required.

Patient not capable of consenting

Where a currently informal patient lacks the capacity to give consent to ECT, there are two main routes available:

- to use the Adults with Incapacity (Scotland) Act 2000 where the patient is not resisting treatment
- to detain the patient under the Mental Health (Scotland) Act 1984 where the patient resists treatment. (The Mental Health Act will also have to be used for compliant, incapable patients who are already detained for another reason.)

The Adults with Incapacity (Scotland) Act 2000 received Royal Assent in May 2000 and Part V, dealing with medical treatment, was implemented in July 2002. The Act applies to people aged 16 and over, and provides for decision making of various sorts, including in relation to medical treatment, for those not capable of making their own decisions. 'Incapable' in the Act is defined as being incapable of acting, or making decisions, or communicating decisions, or understanding decisions, or retaining the memory of decisions, as mentioned in any provision of the Act, by reason of mental disorder or of inability to communicate because of physical disability. The Act is based on general principles, which include the following:

- that the intervention will benefit the adult and that such benefit cannot reasonably be achieved without the intervention
- any intervention must be the least restrictive option in relation to the freedom of the adult, consistent with the purpose of the intervention
- account shall be taken of:
  - the past and present wishes and feelings of the adult so far as they can be ascertained
  - the views of the nearest relative and primary carer of the adult so far as it is reasonable and practicable to do so
  - the views of any guardian, continuing (financial) attorney or welfare attorney of the adult who has powers relating to a proposed intervention and any person whom the sheriff has directed to be consulted
  - the views of any other person appearing to the person responsible for authorising or effecting the intervention to have an interest in the welfare of the adult or in the proposed intervention (where reasonable and practicable to do so).

Section 47 gives authority to the medical practitioner primarily responsible for the medical treatment of an incapable adult, under a 'certificate of incapacity', to give treatment to safeguard or promote physical or mental health so long as it is not treatment requiring the use of force or detention (unless immediately necessary and only for so long as is necessary in the circumstances). In other words, there is a statutory authority to give reasonable treatment to compliant patients incapable of giving consent. Where the patient actively resists or opposes treatment, the clinician should consider the use of the Mental Health Act.

Section 48 of the Act, however, excludes from the statutory authority the giving of any treatment under Part X of the 1984 Act to a patient to whom Part X applies and also special treatment specified by regulations. Regulations have been approved requiring that ECT cannot be given to a patient incapable of consenting to it without a second opinion from a doctor appointed by the Mental Welfare Commission for Scotland. The second-opinion doctor has to complete a prescribed form, set out in schedule 2 of the regulations, which has to be sent to the Commission within 7 days of its issue.

Where the patient is aged 16 or 17, and the RMO is not a specialist in child and adolescent psychiatry, the RMO must obtain a written opinion from such a specialist. The second-opinion doctor appointed by the Commission must be a child and adolescent specialist or have some other relevant experience (e.g. the RMO could be a child and adolescent specialist and the second-opinion doctor a doctor experienced in ECT).

Under the Adults with Incapacity (Scotland) Act 2000, welfare attorneys, welfare guardians and those exercising an intervention order with the appropriate power are able to consent to treatment on behalf of an incapable adult. However, these proxy decision makers cannot consent to special treatments under section 48 of the Act, including ECT. Section 52 of the Act allows anyone with an interest in the personal welfare of the adult, including these proxy decision makers, to appeal a decision regarding a special treatment under section 48 to the sheriff, and from there, with the leave of the sheriff, to the Court of Session. Anyone with an interest can also appeal to the sheriff against a decision of incapacity, under section 14 of the Act, and there are provisions for further appeals to the Sheriff Principal and the Court of Session.

The Code of Practice on Part V of the Act suggests that a section 47 certificate of incapacity is required for treatment under section 48, including ECT, although there is legal argument about whether the Act justifies this statement.

In an emergency, ECT could still be given to an incapable patient under common law, if there is no time to comply with the provisions of the Adults with Incapacity Act. Common law is a body of law built up through court decisions. This area of law is much less well defined in Scotland than it is in England, but there is consensus that it is appropriate in emergencies where there may be a risk to life or limb. The special treatment regulations require that such treatment is reported to the Mental Welfare Commission for Scotland within 7 days.

If treatment is given under common law, good practice dictates consultation with relatives and others with a close interest and the obtaining of an opinion from a consultant colleague, which should be recorded in the notes. The ECT treatment team will wish confirmation that there is lawful authority to proceed with treatment. It may be helpful in this regard for a document to be developed which certifies the patient's incapacity to consent to ECT and the need for it to be given, and records that appropriate processes have been gone through, including a second opinion and consultation with relatives and carers.

Patients subject to emergency detention – sections 24 and 25 Mental Health (Scotland) Act 1984

Emergency detention is excluded from Part X of the Act, so that the authority in section 103 to give treatment in the absence of consent to detained patients, with the qualifications set out in section 98, does not apply. From the point of view of consent to ECT, therefore, a patient subject to emergency detention is in the same position as an informal patient. In view of the urgency of the situation, common law is likely to be the most appropriate authority for treatment of a patient incapable of consent. *As a guide* to the circumstances that may justify treatment being given during emergency detention, without waiting for section 26 to bring in the Part X provisions, the four circumstances defined in section 102 of the Act (outlined below) may be useful. It must be emphasised, however, that *section 102 itself does not apply during emergency detention* but only after Part X has come into effect. Guidance given on treatment under common law in the section above applies in relation to a second opinion, consultation with relatives and so on, and the desirability of having a document to show that the relevant procedures have been followed. If the patient is incapable in relation to consent, regulations under the Adults with Incapacity Act require the reporting of such emergency treatment to the Mental Welfare Commission fpr Scotland within 7 days. Otherwise the Commission requests similar reporting.

Detained patients

Part X of the Mental Health (Scotland) Act 1984 applies to all detained patients except those subject to emergency detention, those taken to a place of safety by the police and restricted patients on conditional discharge. It includes patients on community care orders during the 7-day period of recall to hospital. 'Detained patients' in the context of Part X therefore includes those on section 26 and section 18 and also those admitted to or detained in hospital under the Criminal Procedure (Scotland) Act 1995. In relation to the Criminal Procedure Act, however, it may be that a patient in hospital for *assessment* of his or her mental condition before trial (section 52 of the 1995 Act) or before a decision on disposal (section 200(2)(b)) cannot, without his or her consent, be required to accept treatment for mental disorder until such time as the RMO has satisfied himself or herself that the patient is suffering from a mental disorder of a nature or degree that would warrant admission to hospital under Part IV of the Mental Health (Scotland) Act 1984. It is good practice to record that opinion in writing before the patient is obliged to accept such treatments.

In regulations under section 98 of the 1984 Act, ECT has been specified as a treatment requiring consent or a second opinion in relevant detained patients. Section 98 provides that it is not lawful (except for emergency conditions covered by section 102) to give ECT to a detained patient unless the patient has consented to the treatment and either the RMO or a doctor appointed by the Mental Welfare Commission for Scotland has certified in writing (on form 9) that the patient is capable of understanding the nature, purpose and likely effects of the treatment and has consented to it; or a doctor appointed by the Commission has certified in writing that the patient is not capable of understanding the nature, purpose and likely effects of the treatment or has not consented to it but that, having regard to the likelihood of the treatment alleviating or preventing a deterioration of the patient's condition, the treatment should be given (this is certified on form 10).

Where the patient is able to consent and is consenting to ECT, form 9 is therefore required. The doctor administering the ECT, the anaesthetist and the ECT nurse should expect to see both the ECT consent form and form 9 before giving each treatment. A photocopy of form 9 is acceptable.

Form 9 signifies consent to both ECT and anaesthetic. Although it covers a course of treatment, its existence does not remove the requirement that the need for ECT and consent to it be reconsidered before each proposed treatment. A patient who has given consent can withdraw that consent at any time.

Fluctuating or uncertain consent or consent subject to coercion should not be considered to be valid consent. In any case of doubt, the RMO should seek the opinion of a doctor approved under section 98. Where those administering the ECT have doubts about the patient's consent, this should be brought to the attention of the RMO and appropriate action taken before treatment proceeds. In any discussion about a patient's consent, attention should be paid to any past views of the patient, information from relatives and assessments of members of the multidisciplinary team.

Where the patient is capable of consent but refusing, or incapable of giving or withholding consent, treatment cannot lawfully proceed (unless in emergencies under section 102) unless a doctor appointed by the Mental Welfare Commission for Scotland, under section 9, has visited and examined the patient, discussed the treatment plan with the RMO and signed form 10 to certify agreement with the treatment plan.

The section 98 doctor is asked to agree that the treatment is appropriate for the patient's condition within current responsible professional practice, but it is still a matter for the clinical judgement of those in charge of the patient's treatment whether it is necessary and reasonable to begin or proceed with the course of ECT. The discussion between the section 98 doctor and patient and between the section 98 doctor and RMO should be recorded in the case notes. If there has been any disagreement between the RMO and the section 98 doctor, or a modification of the RMO's treatment plan by the section 98 doctor, this should be clearly recorded. As far as is practicable the patient should be made aware of these discussions and the outcome (normally by the RMO). The ECT treatment team should have sight of the signed form 10 before administering ECT. A photocopied or faxed form is acceptable, but it is not sufficient to have only oral information about the existence of a completed form 10.

The patient's consent may change during the course of ECT along with clinical improvement. Once it is clear that the patient is giving free and informed consent to ECT, form 9 may be substituted for form 10. There is a statutory requirement in section 99 of the 1984 Act to send a report to the Mental Welfare Commission for Scotland when a patient subject to form 10 has his or her detention renewed or discontinued. The Commission also requests section 99 reports at the conclusion of ECT treatment, subject to form 10.

Urgent treatment of detained patients subject to Part X of the 1984 Act

Section 102 provides for the possibility of emergency ECT in circumstances where Part X of the Act applies (e.g. section 26 but not emergency detention) but where it has not been possible to await the arrival of a section 98 doctor. As described above in relation to other UK jurisdictions, four possible circumstances are described in which ECT may be immediately necessary:

- to save the patient's life
- to prevent serious deterioration (not being irreversible)
- to alleviate serious suffering (not being irreversible or hazardous)
- as the minimum necessary intervention to prevent the patient being violent or dangerous to self or others (not being irreversible or hazardous).

As noted above, it has not been stated in statute law that ECT is to be regarded as either intrinsically irreversible or hazardous, but likewise the provisions of section 102 should be used rarely and solely to save the patient's life.

Section 102 treatment should not be given unless a visit by a section 98 doctor has already been requested by the RMO.

In virtually all circumstances it should not be necessary to give more than one or at the most two ECT treatments before the section 98 doctor's visit. Although the section 98 doctor cannot visit until the section 26 detention has started, where urgent ECT is anticipated the Mental Welfare Commission for Scotland will accept a request during preceding emergency detention and begin arrangements for a visit by a section 98 doctor.

Every section 102 treatment must be reported to the Mental Welfare Commission for Scotland in the form suggested in Appendix D at the end of the Mental Health Act Code of Practice (Department of Health & Welsh Office, 1999). This is not a prescribed form, however, and the report can be made by letter.

Good practice would require a second opinion from another consultant, recorded in the case notes, before proceeding with emergency section 102 treatment. It would be of assistance to the ECT treatment team if a document were to be developed that recorded the reason for the treatment under section 102, the making of a request to the Mental Welfare Commission for a visit by a section 98 doctor and the outcome of a local second opinion.

Involvement of relatives of detained patients

Except on behalf of a child considered by the RMO to be too young to give informed consent, and proxy decision makers acting under the Adults with Incapacity (Scotland) Act 2000, no relative may consent to the treatment of another person. It is general good practice, if possible, to gain the cooperation of relatives or close friends in decisions about treatment. The patient should be fully informed that such approaches to relatives or friends are being made. If relatives disagree with the administration of ECT, but the consultant decides to give it, he or she is advised to make a record of the objections and of his or her reasons for proceeding with the treatment.

Future developments

The Scottish Parliament passed the Mental Health (Care and Treatment) (Scotland) Act 2003 in March 2003. Implementation of the bulk of the provisions is expected in April 2005. The new Act is based on stated principles, and the criteria for longer-term compulsory measures are changed, including a new requirement under civil procedure that, because of the mental disorder, the patient's ability to make decisions about medical treatment is significantly impaired. It will also be possible for compulsory measures to be applied without hospitalisation (but this will not be possible for ECT if it has to be given forcibly). Direct entry to short-term detention will be possible, and decisions about short- and long-term compulsory measures will be made by a three-person tribunal rather than the sheriff. The patient will be allowed to select a 'named person' to fulfil some statutory functions previously associated with the nearest relative.

Provisions relating to ECT will be broadly similar to those in the 1984 Act, with the following principal changes:

- The Act will not permit the giving of ECT to a capable and refusing patient, even in emergencies.
- The second-opinion doctor will be known as a 'designated medical practitioner'.
- If the patient is aged under 18, at least one of the RMO or the designated medical practitioner will have to be a child specialist.
- The required certificates will have to state either that the patient is capable of consent and is consenting in writing, or that the patient is incapable of consenting. In either case it will also have to be stated that the treatment is in the patient's best interest, having regard to the likelihood of benefit.
- Where the patient is incapable of consent, the designated medical practitioner will have to consult, where practicable, with the patient, the patient's 'named person' and those principally concerned with the patient's medical treatment.
- If the patient resists or objects to treatment, it will be able to be given only if the designated medical practitioner certifies that treatment is necessary to save life, and/or prevent serious deterioration and/or alleviate serious suffering.
- Certificates, whether the patient is consenting, or incapable of consenting, will be able to be revoked by the Mental Welfare Commission for Scotland.

Republic of Ireland

The Mental Treatment Act 1945 was the relevant legislation at the time of the previous edition of the present book (1995) and it did not deal specifically with treatment and consent. The law on consent is now evolving with the phased implementation of the Mental Health Act 2001, which specified statutory rules for involuntary admission to psychiatric hospital and changes to the legal rights of psychiatric patients. The Act also led to the establishment of the Mental Health Commission in April 2002; the Act specified that the Commission 'shall make rules providing for the use of electro-convulsive therapy and a programme of electro-convulsive therapy shall not be administered to a patient except in accordance with such rules'. This code of practice is not yet available. It will be possible only to outline the general principles of consent to psychiatric treatment and ECT in particular, as specified in the Act.

General principles of consent to psychiatric treatment

Part IV of the Act stipulated that consent means consent in writing, obtained freely, without threats or inducements, where:

- the consultant psychiatrist who is caring for the patient certifies that the patient is capable of understanding the nature, purpose and likely effects of the proposed treatment
- the psychiatrist has given the patient adequate information, in a form and a language that the patient can understand, on the nature, purpose and likely effects of the proposed treatment.

The consent of a patient will be required, except where the consultant psychiatrist considers that the treatment is necessary to safeguard the life of the patient, to restore his or her health, to alleviate his or her condition, or to relieve his or her suffering and the patient is incapable of giving such consent because of his or her mental disorder.

Consent to ECT

Electroconvulsive therapy may not be performed unless the patient gives consent in writing, or the patient is unable or unwilling to give consent and the programme of therapy is approved by the consultant psychiatrist responsible for the care and treatment of the patient, and this is also authorised by another consultant psychiatrist. It is the view of the Commission that for ECT to be performed without the consent of the patient, then the patient would have to fulfil the statutory requirements for involuntary admission to a psychiatric hospital.

Recommendations

- Consent should be obtained only by a registered medical practitioner with adequate knowledge of the nature and effects of ECT. Each ECT clinic should have a policy about who is deemed to be competent to obtain consent in the clinical teams who refer to the clinic.
- The competence of an individual patient to give consent to ECT should always be assessed by a suitably experienced medical practitioner.
- Consent is obtained for a course of treatment, and a maximum number of treatments should be stipulated. Consent should be checked and recorded by the ECT team before each individual treatment.
- A written record must be kept of the assessment of competence and the details of the process of consent or authorisation. Individual patients may have specific questions about the treatment and it would be good practice to record the answers given.
- It is the duty of the referring clinical team to ensure that the proper process for consent or authorisation for treatment is undertaken.
- Liaison between the referring clinical team and the staff in the ECT

clinic is important. In particular, the documentation of the process of consent or authorisation must be available to the staff in the ECT clinic before treatment is undertaken. A photocopy of this documentation would suffice.

- Each doctor or nurse has his or her own ethical and legal duties. The ECT team is not just an agent of the referring team, and has the autonomy to be able to decline to treat a patient. This would be appropriate if the staff in the ECT suite thought that the patient had changed his or her mind about treatment, or the appropriate process of consent or authorisation had not been carried out.
- Other than in Scotland, under the Adults with Incapacity (Scotland) Act 2000, there is no statutory documentation for either the process of authorisation or the use of ECT for people who are incapable of giving informed consent, yet who do not apparently object to treatment. It would be good practice for each ECT clinic to adopt or develop appropriate documentation. Suggested templates are given in Appendix V and Appendix VI.
- It is possible in some circumstances to use existing mental health legislation to administer ECT to a detained patient who is mentally able to give valid informed consent and refuses to consent to ECT. The Special Committee would not regard this as good practice.
- Existing mental health legislation contains provisions to forego the statutory processes of consent to or authorisation of ECT where there is the need for urgent treatment of detained patients. The Special Committee would recommend that these provisions be used solely to save the patient's life.

Contacts

Mental Health Act Commission (England and Wales), Nottingham (0115) 943 7100, www.mhac.trent.nhs.uk
Mental Health Commission for Northern Ireland, Belfast (028) 9065 1157
Mental Welfare Commission for Scotland, Edinburgh (0131) 222 6111, www.mwcscot.org.uk
Mental Health Commission (Republic of Ireland), Dublin 00 353 (1) 636 2400, www.mhcirl.ie

References

Clinical Resource and Audit Group, Working Group on Mental Illness (1997) *Electroconvulsive Therapy: A Good Practice Statement*. Edinburgh: Scottish Executive Department of Health.
Department of Health & Welsh Office (1999) *Mental Health Act 1983: Code of Practice*. Norwich: HMSO.
Freeman, C. P. L., Hendry, J. & Fergusson, G. (2000) *National Audit of Electroconvulsive Therapy in Scotland. Final Report*. Available at www.sean.org.uk/report/report00.php.

Jones, R. M. (1999) Mental Health Act Manual (6th edn), pp. 240–241. London: Sweet & Maxwell.

Mental Welfare Commission for Scotland (1999) *Guidance on Consent Issues for ECT Coordinators*. Available at www.sean.org.uk/report/report23.php.

Mental Welfare Commission for Scotland (2003) *Annual Report 2002–2003*. Available at www.mwcscot.org.uk/annualreports.htm.

Further source

British Medical Association (1995) *Assessment of Mental Capacity: Guidance for Doctors and Lawyers*. London: BMA.

Appendices

How does ECT work?[*]

Ian C. Reid

The use of ECT is often criticised on the basis that the mode of action of the treatment is unknown. It is true that the convulsive treatments were developed in the context of ideas about the nature of mental illness and its relationship to epilepsy that are now known to be incorrect. The place of ECT in contemporary psychiatry is founded instead on empirical demonstrations of safety and effectiveness. None the less, a great deal is known about the effects of ECT in the central nervous system (CNS) and that knowledge base continues to grow. An understanding of the action of ECT can tell us a great deal about the pathophysiology of the conditions it so effectively treats, and could ultimately lead to its replacement with more effective therapies. It is precisely because the pathophysiology of mood disorder is incompletely understood that explanations of how the treatment works must remain provisional. There are many noble examples of this situation throughout the history of medicine. The use of lime juice to prevent scurvy was practised a century before the discovery of vitamin C. Similarly, the successful use of cowpox in vaccination against smallpox was conducted long before viruses were identified and understood. Indeed, a comprehensive explanation for the complex actions of aspirin is only now beginning to emerge.

Like the chemical antidepressants, ECT is known to modulate monoamine systems in the brain such as the serotonergic and noradrenergic pathways. It enhances the activity of dopaminergic systems, which explains some of its effectiveness not only in depressive disorder but also in Parkinson's disease. It has potent anticonvulsant properties, which it shares with the anticonvulsant drugs now used in the treatment and prophylaxis of bipolar disorder. It has powerful effects on excitatory amino acid systems, which are increasingly implicated in psychosis. These wide-ranging actions go some way to explaining the

---

[*]This contribution was commissioned from Professor Reid in response to practitioners who had asked for the inclusion of a short summary for teaching purposes.

effectiveness of ECT in a range of different conditions, such as depressive disorder, mania and schizophrenia. Although ECT has effects on many systems in the brain, the individual effects on neurotransmitter systems may be more specific and focused than those induced by chemical antidepressants.

Recent studies in animals suggest that ECT has potent effects in bolstering neuronal survival, in sharp contradiction to the commonly held but unfounded view that ECT must somehow harm neurons. It even promotes the production of new neurons and new neural processes in areas of the brain known to be involved in cognitive and emotional function. In common with chemical antidepressant treatments, ECT enhances the expression of a neuroprotective protein, brain-derived neurotrophic factor (BDNF), which antagonises the neurotoxic effects of stress on the brain. These are important findings, because it is increasingly appreciated that chronic depression is associated with atrophy of brain structures in the frontal and temporal lobes, and ECT may act to arrest or even reverse these degenerative effects.

Further reading

Reid, I. C. & Stewart, C. A. (2001) How antidepressants work: new perspectives on the pathophysiology of depressive disorder. *British Journal of Psychiatry*, **178**, 299–303.

Information for users and carers

As noted in the Introduction, a College factsheet will be prepared separately by the College as a public information exercise and involve representatives of users, carers, other professional organisations and the voluntary sector. In the meantime, it may be helpful for readers to know that in 1996 the Manic Depression Fellowship and the Scottish Association for Mental Health jointly published an information booklet, *ECT: Your Questions Answered*, which is available electronically on the website of the Scottish ECT Audit Network (www.sean.org.uk/ectqu/ectqu0.php). Other resources for patients, carers, and lay people are available electronically from the website www.sean.org.uk.

Out-patient ECT: example protocol and additional information for out-patients

Out-patient protocol

Before out-patient ECT, an appointment should be arranged for the patient to attend the ward to have all the necessary investigations carried out. Information on ECT should be given to patients before they attend this appointment.

The investigations should be done before the day of treatment, to allow results to be obtained and any concerns or problems to be dealt with and passed on to the ECT team.

Where possible, the patient and his or her carer should be given the opportunity to discuss the treatment and go over any concerns or worries they may have with an appropriate person on the day they attend this appointment. If treatment is to go ahead, then a letter informing the patient's general practitioner should be sent.

The patient should be advised to attend the ward at a specific time on the day of treatment. A responsible adult must collect the patient and a responsible adult must be with him or her that night, if the patient returns home the same day. The patient and the principal carer should be asked to read and sign a disclaimer form to confirm that they are aware of all important information.

The patient may remain in hospital overnight after treatment, but if this is not necessary should remain in the ward at least until a specified time, when he or she should be seen by a doctor to establish whether or not the patient is mentally and physically fit to leave. If so, this should be recorded in the hospital records. If the doctor feels that the patient is not medically fit to be discharged from hospital, but the patient insists on going home, then the patient should be asked to sign an 'against medical advice' discharge form. If the doctor feels that the patient is not psychiatrically fit to be discharged, compulsory admission under the appropriate Mental Health Act may be indicated.

If the patient is discharged, he or she should be reminded not to drive for at least 24 hours after treatment. (He/she will not be insured to do so.)

No patient should leave either on the day of treatment or the next day until a medical examination has been performed and the fitness for discharge has been recorded in the hospital records. This is not the responsibility of the nursing staff.

All patients receiving out-patient ECT must be reviewed at least as often as in-patients. The ECT team must be informed of any significant changes.

Should the patient develop suicidal ideation during the course of treatment, then serious consideration should be given to admission to hospital for the remainder of the course of ECT.

At the end of the course of treatment, a letter should again be sent to the general practitioner detailing the treatment and outcome.

Out-patient ECT information

Name:
Date:
Unit number:
Ward:
Consultant:
Key worker:
Ward doctor:
Ward telephone number:

Today you received electroconvulsive therapy. This involved a general anaesthetic; therefore you should not do any of the following for at least the next 24 hours:

- drive any type of vehicle
- operate machinery or electrical appliances
- consume alcohol.

You should have another responsible adult to remain with you for the first 24 hours after treatment.

If you suffer any serious side-effects, then contact your own general practitioner in the first instance and pass on the information on this sheet.

If you have any concerns relating to your treatment or develop a cold or physical illness, then contact the ward that organised your ECT treatment. The information will be passed on to your hospital doctor.

The evening before your next treatment, please remember not to eat any food after midnight, and take the tablets or medicines only as agreed with your hospital doctor.

Example of a consent form

Name of hospital

Patient agreement to electroconvulsive therapy (ECT)

Patient details (or pre-printed label)

Patient's surname/family name:

Patient's first names:

Date of birth:

Consultant psychiatrist:

NHS number (or other identifier):

• Male   • Female

Special requirements :
(e.g. other language/other communication method)

To be retained in patient's notes

Patient's name:

A course of bilateral/unilateral electroconvulsive therapy up to a maximum of ... treatments.
(This section must be completed. If a number is not stated, then treatment will not be given.)

Statement of health professional (to be filled in by: ...)

I have explained the procedure to the patient. In particular, I have explained:

The intended benefits:
- improvement of depression
- other (specify):

Serious/frequently occurring risks:
- memory loss (possibly permanent)
- post-treatment confusion

Transient side-effects
- headache
- muscle aches
- nausea
- 'muzzy-headedness'
- fatigue

I have also discussed what the procedure is likely to involve, the benefits and risks of any available alternative treatments (including no treatment) and any particular concerns of this patient.

- The following leaflet has been provided – *ECT Information Booklet*

This procedure will involve:
- general anaesthesia
- muscle relaxation

Signed:
Date :
Name (PRINT):
Job title:

Contact details (if patient wishes to discuss options later) ... **(via secretary)**

Statement of interpreter (where appropriate)

I have interpreted the information above to the patient to the best of my ability and in a way in which I believe s/he can understand.

Signed:
Date:
Name (PRINT):

Copy accepted by patient: yes/no (please ring)

Statement of patient

Patient identifier/label:
Please read this form carefully. You should already have your own copy of page 2 and an information booklet that describes the intended benefits and frequently occurring risks of ECT. If not, you will be offered a copy now. If you have any further questions, do ask – we are here to help you. You have the right to change your mind **at any time**, including **after you have signed this form.**

I agree to the procedure and course of treatment described on this form.

I understand that you cannot give me a guarantee that a particular person will perform the procedure. The person will, however, have appropriate experience.

I understand that I will have the opportunity to discuss the details of anaesthesia with an anaesthetist before the procedure, unless the urgency of my situation prevents this.

I understand that any procedure in addition to those described on this form will be carried out only if it is necessary to save my life or to prevent serious harm to my health.

I have been told about additional procedures that may become necessary during my treatment. I have listed below any procedures that **I do not wish to be carried out** without further discussion:

Patient's signature:
Date:
Name (PRINT):

A witness should sign below if the patient is unable to sign but has indicated his or her consent:

Signature:
Date:
Name (PRINT):

Important notes: (tick if applicable)
- See also advance directive/living will (e.g. Jehovah's Witness form)

Confirmation or withdrawal of consent

To be completed by a health professional each time the patient attends for the procedure, if the patient has signed the form in advance.

Patient name:

On behalf of the team treating the patient, I have confirmed with the patient that s/he has no further questions and wishes the procedure to go ahead. I have explained that the patient may withdraw consent at any time.

Signed:
Date:
Name (PRINT):
Job title:

The form will have sufficient such entries to cover the entire course of treatment.

Patient has withdrawn consent

Ask patient to sign and date here:

If consent withdrawn, date of last treatment:

Guidance to health professionals

To be read in conjunction with consent policy.

What a consent form is for

This form documents the patient's agreement to go ahead with the investigation or treatment you have proposed. It is not a legal waiver – if patients, for example, do not receive enough information on which to base their decision, then the consent may not be valid, even though the form has been signed. Patients are also entitled to change their mind after signing the form, if they retain capacity to do so. The form should act as an *aide-memoire* to health professionals and patients, by providing a checklist of the kind of information patients should be offered, and by enabling the patient to have a written record of the main points discussed. In no way, however, should the written information provided for the patient be regarded as a substitute for face-to-face discussions with the patient.

The law on consent

See the Department of Health's *Reference Guide to Consent for Examination or Treatment* for a comprehensive summary of the law on consent.*

Who can give consent

Everyone aged 16 or more is presumed to be competent to give consent for themselves, unless the opposite is demonstrated. If a child under the age of 16 has 'sufficient understanding and intelligence to enable him or her to understand fully what is proposed', then he or she will be competent to give consent for himself or herself. Young people aged 16 and 17, and legally 'competent' younger children, may therefore sign this form for themselves, but may like a parent to countersign as well. If the child is not able to give consent for himself or herself, someone with parental responsibility may do so on their behalf and a separate form is available for this purpose. Even where a child is able to give consent for himself or herself, you should always involve those with parental responsibility in the child's care, unless the child specifically asks you not to do so. If a patient is mentally competent to give consent but is physically unable to sign a form, you should complete this form as usual, and ask an independent witness to confirm that the patient has given consent orally or non-verbally.

---

*Available at www.dh.gov.uk/PublicationsAndStatistics/Publications/
PublicationsPolicyAndGuidance/PublicationsPolicyAndGuidanceArticle/fs/
en?CONTENT_ID=4006757&chk=snmdw8.

When not to use this form

If the patient is 18 or over and is not legally competent to give consent, you should use form 4 (form for adults who are unable to consent to investigation or treatment) instead of this form. Patients will not be legally competent to give consent if:

- they are unable to comprehend and retain information material to the decision
- they are unable to weigh and use this information in coming to a decision.

You should always take all reasonable steps (for example involving more specialist colleagues) to support patients in making their own decision, before concluding that they are unable to do so.

Relatives **cannot** be asked to sign this form on behalf of an adult who is not legally competent to consent for himself or herself.

Information

Information about what the treatment will involve, its benefits and risks (including side-effects and complications) and the alternatives to the particular procedure proposed is crucial for patients when making up their minds. The courts have stated that patients should be told about 'significant risks which would affect the judgement of a reasonable patient'. 'Significant' has not been legally defined, but the General Medical Council requires doctors to tell patients about 'serious or frequently occurring' risks. In addition, if patients make clear they have particular concerns about certain kinds of risk, you should make sure they are informed about these risks, even if they are very slight. You should always answer questions honestly. Sometimes, patients may make it clear that they do not want to have any information about the options, but want you to decide on their behalf. In such circumstances, you should do your best to ensure that the patient receives at least very basic information about what is proposed. Where information is refused, you should document this on the form or in the patient's notes.

Incapacitated compliant patients – a suggested template for authorisation

ECT for incapacitated compliant patients

I ... of ...

and being the ... (state status in respect of patient's treatment)

confirm that ... of ...

requires a course of ECT in order to prevent a deterioration or ensure an improvement in his/her physical or mental health.

I also confirm that:

- the patient lacks the capacity to fully consent to this procedure because of his/her physical or psychiatric condition

- the patient has not indicated in word or deed a lack of compliance with other current aspects of his/her treatment (including in-patient hospital stay).

I have had appropriate discussions with the patient's carers/relatives.

Date:
Signed:

NB – this Appendix will not be relevant in Scotland (see Chapter 20).

Emergency treatment – a suggested template for authorisation

ECT given in an emergency

I ... of ...

certify that ... of ...

requires emergency treatment with ECT. The reason for this is:

I confirm that the treatment has been deemed appropriate by ... who is a consultant psychiatrist of ...

I also confirm that I have consulted the appropriate relatives and/or carers of the patient.

Date:
Signed:

Note: This authorisation will be valid for no more than 7 days and will authorise no more than 2 treatment sessions.

Nursing guidelines for ECT

Linda Cullen, RMN RGN

The responsibilities of the ECT nurse have increased over recent years, making this role pivotal within the ECT team. This appendix contains guidelines for good practice, a description of the main responsibilities of the ECT nurse, escort nurse and nurse in charge of recovery. An example of a job description for an ECT nurse is included.

The ECT nurse

The nurse responsible for the running of the ECT clinic should be a registered nurse who is a minimum of a 'G' grade or equivalent. He or she should be a designated person who is primarily employed as an ECT nurse or seconded to this role (it should not be left to a nurse drafted in from a ward who is available on the day of treatment). There should be a fully trained deputy who regularly attends ECT and is available to provide cover for the clinic during leave of the nurse in charge.

The nurse should have protected time to carry out all the duties required and should not be expected to be covering a ward or other responsibilities on the days of treatment. The sessional time should be adequate to allow the ECT nurse to carry out the following areas of responsibility:

- spending time with patients and relatives in order to provide support and information
- liaising with the prescribing teams and ECT team
- assisting in treatment sessions
- updating of protocols and policies
- performing audit and risk assessment
- training (staff and personal)

These guidelines were endorsed by the Royal College of Nursing in February 2004.
The appendix includes contributions from the Glasgow ECT Nurses Forum and North West ECT Nurses Group.

- administration
- maintenance of equipment and environment
- ordering and stocking of treatment suite.

The ECT nurse should have a good working knowledge of the ECT procedure, complications and possible side-effects, both common and rare (see also 'Staff training and personal development', below). He or she will also need to be aware of the required routine investigations and the significance of their results.

The ECT nurse is best placed to meet with patients to discuss the procedure and any concerns, as he or she will be in possession of up-to-date information. Both written and verbal information on ECT should be given to all patients and specific day-case information should be given to those attending for day-case ECT. This opportunity can be used to show the patient around the ECT clinic if appropriate. Meeting the ECT nurse before the first treatment session can help to reduce the patient's anxieties (as the patient may recognise a familiar face when attending the clinic) and also provides better continuity of care.

Before the treatment session

Before a treatment session, the ECT nurse should:

- liaise with wards and prescribing team to ensure that the information on the patient is up to date and all relevant investigations have been carried out before treatment (and the ECT nurse should pass on any significant results to the other members of the ECT team)
- organise and schedule appointments for treatments for both in-patients and day-case patients to ensure smooth running of the treatment session and minimise waiting time for patients
- provide information and support for patients and their relatives (where possible)
- ensure ward-based staff are aware of preparation of patients (routine investigations, required accompanying documentation, etc. – a protocol containing all this information should be available to all the wards that are likely to send patients for ECT)
- coordinate the ECT team and keep them informed of times, patient numbers, patient details and any other significant information.

During a treatment session

During a treatment session the ECT nurse should:

- carry out and record routine pre-ECT nursing checks on patients when they attend for treatment, or delegate this task to a suitably trained assistant or deputy

- check patients' legal status and consent and that all relevant documentation is present (e.g. case notes, consent form, legal documents)
- ensure that any concerns or issues arising from nursing checks on patients are passed on to the relevant members of the ECT team (e.g. changes to consent, legal status, medication, physical condition)
- provide support and reassurance for patients while in they are in the clinic
- ensure the safety and comfort of the patient throughout the treatment
- introduce the ECT team to the patient
- carry out any required preparation of patient (e.g. applying the electroencephalogram electrodes)
- update the ECT team on a patient's condition if that patient has had previous treatment (side-effects, response to treatment, etc.)
- assist the psychiatrist with the timing of the duration of the seizure by use of the chosen method (e.g. stopwatch, Hamilton cuff technique or EEG monitoring, in accordance with local protocols)
- observe the patient throughout treatment and record observations such as oxygen saturation, blood pressure, heart rate, seizure duration and quality, EEG monitoring, time to spontaneous breathing and any other significant events (unless done by the anaesthetist, anaesthetic assistant or psychiatrist, as agreed by local protocols)
- assist with placing patient in recovery position prior to transfer to recovery area
- escort the patient through to the recovery area and ensure relevant information is passed on to the nurse in charge of recovery (the anaesthetist should pass on any specific instructions for the recovery to nurse in charge of recovery, and any drugs, intravenous fluids or oxygen to be administered should have a written pre-scription)
- prepare the treatment room for the next patient (change disposable equipment, clean or change electrodes, etc.)
- discuss the treatment of the next patient with the team before that patient enters, which will include checking and setting the treatment dose with the psychiatrist (this should be checked again verbally before the treatment button is pressed).

The nurse should be fully conversant with the use of the particular ECT machine in the clinic and should be able to carry out the self-test procedure in accordance with local protocol. The ECT nurse should not administer the treatment but should assist the psychiatrist by operating the controls on the fascia of the ECT machine while the psychiatrist applies the electrodes. The nurse should check the dose (which should be set by the psychiatrist) and confirm verbally with the psychiatrist before pressing the treat button. This should be done in accordance with a locally agreed protocol.

There should be a minimum of two trained nurses in the treatment room during the administration of the treatment (this may be the ECT nurse and the escorting nurse).

A suitably trained anaesthetic assistant should be present during the treatment, in accordance with the guidelines laid down by the Association of Anaesthetists of Great Britain and Ireland (2002) (e.g. an operating department practitioner/assistant, or a nurse with appropriate training). (This can be the ECT nurse provided he or she has received adequate training and it is in agreement with the ECT anaesthetist and local protocol.)

The ECT nurse should have knowledge of:

- the actions required in the event of a medical emergency (e.g. suxamethonium apnoea, malignant hyperpyrexia, laryngospasm) (local protocols on these topics should be available to all the team)
- the drugs used for ECT, their appropriate doses, potential side-effects and the appropriate treatment of those side-effects
- dosing policy
- the local protocol for termination of prolonged seizures (and have the required equipment and drugs readily available to anaesthetist).

After treatment

After treatment the ECT nurse should ensure that day-case patients are not discharged until fully recovered. (It is good practice for the ECT nurse to have them seen by a doctor before agreeing their discharge from their care.) Day-case patients must be collected by a responsible adult and should not be allowed to leave alone or drive a vehicle. (Patients and the person collecting them should be reminded of this before they leave and advised to consult the specific day-case information they were given at the outset of treatment.)

It is advantageous (where possible) to be able to visit ECT patients in the afternoon following their treatment as this allows the ECT nurse to follow up patients, which gives the nurse an opportunity to observe any side-effects and address any concerns or anxieties patients may have. It also provides better continuity of care, and helps to build a more therapeutic relationship between the patient and the ECT nurse, helping to reduce patients' anxieties in consequent treatments.

The ECT nurse should provide feedback to both the prescribing team and ECT team, and ensure that all relevant documentation has been completed.

Administrative duties

The ECT nurse should:

- be well versed in local and national guidelines and should regularly update protocols and policies accordingly
- complete ECT records on each patient's visit to the ECT clinic in accordance with the local protocol
- carry out regular audits of practice and patient care.

Maintenance/environment

The ECT nurse should:

- ensure the ECT clinic is a safe environment for both patients and staff
- organise regular maintenance of equipment and the environment and keep detailed records on this
- carry out and keep updated risk assessments within the unit and take action to address any issues of concern
- be familiar with the use of all the equipment in the ECT clinic
- check expiry dates on all disposable equipment and order required stock
- check expiry dates on all routine and emergency drugs and order as appropriate.

Staff training and personal development

The ECT nurse should:

- have a good knowledge of possible drug interactions and side-effects, and the required treatment
- undertake regular training in basic life support and preferably immediate life support or advanced life support, to meet the requirements of local protocols
- provide training and support to escort and ward nurses
- have a reasonable level of training and experience of airway management (this should be regularly updated)
- possess a good working knowledge of legal status and consent (e.g. the implications and requirements to be met)
- organise teaching sessions for students and new staff
- attend a Royal College of Psychiatrists' training day or other appropriate ECT training to update their knowledge (adequate time and financial support to attend this type of training should be provided by management, as it is important that practice and standards are regularly updated).

Role of the escorting nurse

The escorting nurse should *always* be a trained nurse – without exception.

Each patient should be individually escorted. To this end, adequate staffing levels should be agreed with management and provision made to meet the need on ECT treatment days. This may require staggering of treatments to ensure adequate staffing levels from wards and this should be arranged at local level between wards and the ECT team.

The escorting nurse should have:

- up-to-date training in basic life support and be competent in its practice
- a good knowledge of the ECT process, especially the possible side-effects (both common and rare) and the nursing actions required in the event of their occurrence
- familiarity with the clinic environment, especially the location of emergency equipment (in the use of which the nurse should be trained and competent).

Escorting nurses should know the patients they are escorting and be aware of their legal status, consent and any possible medical complications. They should carry out pre-ECT nursing checks at ward level to ensure patients are properly prepared and all the relevant documentation is available to take to the ECT clinic. These checks should include recording of patient's pulse and blood pressure in order that the ECT team has a baseline set of observations. They should ensure the safe keeping of patients' valuables or any prosthesis (although any prosthesis should not be removed until immediately before treatment at the ECT clinic).

The escorting nurse should check the patient in recovery in accordance with local protocols, which may include determining heart rate, oxygen saturation, blood pressure, level of responsiveness and level of orientation. He or she should ensure the patient's safety within the recovery room, and remain with the patient and provide support and orientation throughout the whole process until such time as the patient is suitably recovered, and escort him or her back to the ward. (In the case of day-case patients the nurse should remain with the patient until such time that he or she is returned to the ward or a suitably trained person is available to take over care or the patient is collected by a responsible adult.)

Role of the nurse in charge of recovery

The guidelines below are in accordance with recommendations of the Association of Anaesthetists of Great Britain and Ireland (2002).

There should be one trained nurse with overall responsibility in the treatment room. This should not be the ECT nurse or one of the escorting nurses. There should be a minimum of two trained nurses in the recovery room at all times during the recovery process. At all times at least one person in the recovery room must hold an up-to-date certificate in advanced life support (or equivalent). The nurse in charge of recovery is probably the most appropriate person to be this person.

The nurse in charge of recovery should:

- have a good knowledge of the ECT process, especially the possible side-effects (both common and rare) and the nursing actions required in the event of their occurrence
- be familiar with the ECT clinic and location of emergency equipment and be trained and competent in its use
- be competent in all aspects of basic life support and immediate life support
- have received training in recovery procedures, airway management and so on, and be up to date and competent in their practice (this can usually be arranged through the local theatre department)
- receive a hand-over from the anaesthetist with regard to each patient and any specific instructions given – any intravenous fluids, drugs or oxygen therapy must be properly prescribed and this information should in turn be passed on to the trained nurse escort with the patient
- provide a safe environment for both staff and patients while in the recovery area
- supervise the care of the patient in the most acute stages of recovery and be available to address any concerns of escorting nurses regarding their patients
- alert the anaesthetist to any concerns or adverse events during recovery
- orientate patients to their situation and environment
- complete any relevant documentation before the patient returns to ward or home
- ensure that patients are not discharged back to the ward until fully recovered, with their observations stable (the anaesthetist should either discharge patients from recovery or provide the nurse in charge of recovery with strict criteria for discharge)
- ensure that day-case patients are fully recovered before they leave, that they do so in the company of a responsible adult and that they are aware that they are not permitted to drive
- remind all day-case patients of the specific instructions for day-case treatment and advise them to refer to the day-case information sheet they were given at outset of treatment.

Example of a job description for an ECT nurse

1. Job details

Title:	ECT Coordinator
Salary/scale:	G grade or equivalent
Responsible to:	Senior Nurse Manager
Service population:	Patients (in-patient or community) who require ECT

2. Job purpose

As a member of the clinical team within this area of specialist practice, you will provide professional advice, support, direction and supervision to nursing staff, as well as other staff new to the working area. You will be actively involved in maintaining and improving practice standards within your area of responsibility and raising awareness of all staff of any developments. You will provide a professional and education resource to nurse managers and clinical directors and have a remit to colleagues throughout mental health services and users to ensure that a consistent approach to service provision is maintained. You will maintain professional standards and promote research and development within the department.

3. Area-specific responsibilities

- Provide guidance, support and expertise relating to patient care in the psychological and physical preparation for ECT.
- Offer full knowledge and understanding of informed consent and its application to patients' circumstances and needs.
- Knowledge of Mental Health (Scotland) Act 1984 legislation in relation to ECT, as well as the wider context.
- Ensure effective communication between all disciplines involved in ECT delivery and good customer and public relations within the hospital, the trust and the community.
- Anaesthetic support practice and knowledge which encompasses:
  - suitable preparation of the environment
  - pre-treatment clinical assessment and work-up
  - anaesthetic circuits and other equipment available within the treatment area
  - all related pharmacology, including induction agents, depolarising muscle relaxants and emergency drugs
  - identification of a normal ECG and recognition of arrhythmias and their treatment
  - identification of the importance of baseline recordings and how they are affected by anaesthetic agents
  - oxygenation needs before, during and after treatment
  - care of and protection of the unconscious patient

- identification of monitoring needs and the operation of equipment/procedures related to this function
- post-anaesthetic care, complete recovery criteria and the principles involved
- basic and advanced life support techniques.
- Ensure the smooth implementation of all organisation/operational issues related to this professional service.
- Full knowledge of contraindications, indications and adverse effects of ECT and able to communicate this information effectively.
- Assess/evaluate immediate and longer-term response to ECT.
- Develop internal audit mechanisms in liaison with other disciplines and the SEAN group (Scottish ECT Audit Network, 2000).
- Actively participate in research/further study for the improvement of care and ECT delivery, as well as support other staff involved.
- Provide an annual report for service managers to include statistical details, developmental achievements and future aims of the service.
- Provide ongoing enhancement of training/induction programmes for all staff.
- Policy development, implementation and systematic review.
- Implement and support clinical development plans for nursing staff within your department.

4. Generic responsibilities

- Liaise with Senior Nurse Manager in the identification of staffing requirements and agree appropriate actioning.
- Ensure annual leave is balanced and allocated appropriately and efficiently.
- Monitor sickness/absence and review information with Senior Nurse Manager.
- Adhere to local policies with regard to reporting accidents and incidents and ensure matters are fully discussed with appropriate staff.
- Establish and maintain an effective and facilitative communication system which will maximise the dissemination of information.

5. Key result areas

UKCC – Scope of Professional Practice
Scottish Office guidelines
Mental Health Act legislation
Mental Welfare Commission good practice guidelines
Special Committee on ECT
National Audit Project
Royal College of Anaesthetists' guidelines
User group forums

Royal College of Nursing – ECT practice guidelines
Clinical supervision – networking with other ECT coordinators regularly

6. Review of work and appraisal

Within 8 weeks of taking up this post you will, with your line manager, agree and record personal objectives consistent with organisational and professional requirements.

At mutually agreed intervals, performance will be appraised, taking previously agreed objectives and personal development into account.

7. Job description agreement

Job holder's signature:
Date:

Line manager's signature:
Date:
Line manager's title:

Sources

Association of Anaesthetists of Great Britain and Ireland (2002) *Immediate Post-anaesthetic Recovery*. London: Association of Anaesthetists of Great Britain and Ireland.
Clinical Resource and Audit Group, Working Group on Mental Illness (1997) *Electroconvulsive Therapy (ECT): A Good Practice Statement*. Edinburgh: Scottish Office.
Scottish ECT Audit Network (2000) www.sean.org

An example of a stimulus dosing protocol

ECT Department, Royal Edinburgh Hospital

Stimulus dosing protocol for Ectron Series 5 ECT machine

General aims

- The seizure threshold should be routinely measured by an empirical titration method. An operational definition of the seizure threshold is 'the minimum amount of electrical charge (in mC) that will induce a classical generalised tonic–clonic convulsion at the first or second treatment in a course of ECT'.
- The aim is for the dose of electrical charge in subsequent treatments to be clearly supra-threshold – to maximise the efficacy of treatment – and yet avoid dosages that are grossly supra-threshold – because this contributes unnecessarily to the cognitive adverse effects of treatment.
- The only exception to these general aims is where treatment is started in an emergency to save life. It is then not desirable to initiate treatment with a threshold dose and it is better to estimate the seizure threshold and treat with a supra-threshold dose to maximise the therapeutic effect. In these rare indications, it is necessary to consult the supervising psychiatrist to discuss how to initiate treatment for the individual patient.

Titration of seizure threshold

Patients not taking anti-epileptic drugs

The first stimulation at the first treatment will routinely be 50 mC. If the necessary convulsion is not induced after 20 seconds, stimulation will be repeated with a dose of 75 mC. If the necessary convulsion is not induced after the second stimulation, the third stimulation should be increased to 175 mC. (Very few patients free of anti-epileptic drugs will fail to have a convulsion with a dose of 175 mC at the first session of ECT.) Assuming that 175 mC led to the necessary convulsion at the first treatment, the titration procedure can be continued at the second treatment session by applying 100 mC at the first stimulation, and, if the necessary convulsion is not induced, increasing the dose to 125 mC at the second stimulation. If the necessary convulsion is still not induced, then the third stimulation should be 225 mC for bilateral ECT and 600 mC for unilateral ECT. (The seizure threshold must be at least 150 mC.)

See the worked example below and also note 1.

Patients taking anti-epileptic drugs

The absolute values and range of stimulation at the first treatment should be higher than those applicable to patients not taking such drugs: that is, 100 mC, 200 mC and 300 mC. At the second treatment, the titration process can continue between the lower stimulation that did not lead to a convulsion and the higher stimulation that did.

Calculation of the seizure threshold

Ideally, the dose that did not induce the necessary convulsion will be only 25 mC less than the dose that did. Although the actual seizure threshold will lie between these two values, it is sufficient to take the upper value as the seizure threshold. (See note 2.)

Dosing strategy

Once the seizure threshold has been established at the first or second treatment, then the dose must be increased at the next treatment session to exceed the threshold as follows:

* For bilateral ECT, the dose should exceed the seizure threshold by 50% (i.e. be 1.5 times) the seizure threshold.
* For unilateral ECT, the dose should be four times the seizure threshold.
* The only exception to these general rules is the patient who displayed the necessary convulsion with only 50 mC, and is to be treated by unilateral ECT. It will be sufficient to increase the dose by only three times. (The minimum dose from the machine is 50 mC and it could be that the initial seizure threshold is as low as 25 mC in unilateral ECT.)

Seizure monitoring

- It is the responsibility of the treating doctor to time the length of the generalised convulsion. The stopwatch should be started at the end of electrical stimulation and stopped at the end of generalised (i.e. bilateral) clonic activity. This time should be recorded on the prescription sheet. If isolated clonic activity in a limb continues beyond generalised activity, this time should also be recorded.
- There is no simple relationship between the length of the convulsion and the therapeutic efficacy of treatment; nevertheless, it is important to time the convulsion because it means the treating psychiatrist ensures that a generalised tonic–clonic convulsion has been induced.

Adjusting the dose throughout a course of treatment

This may be indicated for the following reasons:

- Repeated ECT can lead to a rise in the seizure threshold, and a dose that initially induced the necessary convulsion may fail to do so later in the course of treatment. A higher dose will therefore be required. It is sometimes said that a progressive shortening in convulsion length over a course of treatment means that the seizure threshold is rising; this is not invariable. In such a situation it is important that the ECT team finds out from the referring team how well the patient is progressing with treatment; if improvement is absent or slight, then it may be entirely reasonable to increase the dose.
- The initial dosing strategy brings about only slight or no clinical improvement. Doses up to 150% above (i.e. 2.5 times) the seizure threshold may be indicated in bilateral ECT, and doses up to six times the seizure threshold in unilateral ECT.
- Significant treatment-emergent cognitive adverse effects such as prolonged disorientation after treatment may be an indication to reduce the electrical dose. Please discuss the management of such adverse effects on an individual basis with the supervising psychiatrist.

See also note 3.

Failure to induce a convulsion

The protocol has already covered how to proceed if stimulation does not lead to a convulsion during titration of the seizure threshold. Later on in a course of treatment, stimulation may fail to induce a convulsion if there has been a marked rise in the seizure threshold (see above) or because of a change in a variable that independently alters the seizure threshold (e.g. the prescription of an anti-epileptic drug or a change in anaesthetic technique). It is essential to repeat stimulation with a higher dose. If it would be desirable to establish the new, higher seizure threshold, then a small increase in dose will be appropriate, that is, 25–50 mC. But if the patient is severely ill, it is not desirable to treat with a dose close to threshold; it is better to estimate that the new seizure threshold is 25–50 mC higher than the dose that did not lead to a convulsion, and then use this estimate to calculate the dose for restimulation as per the dosing strategy above.

Termination of a prolonged convulsion

A prolonged convulsion is one that lasts 2 minutes or more, and should be terminated immediately, either by a further dose of induction agent or by intravenous administration of a benzodiazepine drug. Prolonged convulsions must be terminated promptly in consultation with the anaesthetist. Once a convulsion of, say, 90 seconds has been observed, then it would be wise for the treating psychiatrist and anaesthetist to express a preference for which treatment will be used to terminate convulsive activity and to prepare such treatment.

A worked example (bilateral ECT, no anti-epileptic)

Treatment	Stimulation	Convulsion	Comments
1	50 mC	0	
	75 mC	0	
	175 mC	41 s generalised convulsion	The seizure threshold lies between 76 and 174 mC
2	100 mC	19 s generalised convulsion	The seizure threshold lies between 76 and 100 mC. Taken as 100 mC
3	150 mC	45 s generalised convulsion	Dose = seizure threshold + 50%. The convulsion induced by supra-threshold stimulation is longer
4	150 mC	43 s generalised convulsion	
5	150 mC	38 s generalised convulsion	
6	150 mC	19 s generalised convulsion	

Note reduction in length of convulsion at sixth treatment. Discuss with referring team whether or not there is an indication to increase dose.

The protocol may be updated by further experience or research findings.

Note 1

The question is sometimes asked how best to proceed when a patient has been treated previously by ECT. Research evidence is scanty, but as an operational policy the following is suggested. If it is 3 months or more since the patient last had ECT, this should be ignored and titration proceed as per normal. If between 3 months and 2 weeks, the titration should be as for patients on anti-epileptic drugs. If the interval is 2 weeks or less, dosing should continue as if the patient were continuing with the same course of ECT.

Note 2

Before deciding how to dose the patient, you must ask yourself what you believe the patient's seizure threshold to be on that day and before you stimulate the patient. It may be helpful to record the seizure threshold on the form (e.g. ST = 75 mC).

Note 3

Both inadequate clinical improvement and treatment-emergent cognitive adverse effects may affect the choice of electrode placement. Patients who do not recover from depressive illness with high-dose unilateral ECT may subsequently recover with moderate-dose bilateral ECT. Prolonged disorientation is much less of a risk in unilateral ECT.

Allan I. F. Scott
January 2005

An example of a protocol for continuation ECT

Continuation ECT should be considered for patients who have relapsing or refractory depression which has previously responded well to ECT but for whom standard pharmacological and psychological continuation treatment is ineffective or inappropriate. Such patients might include:

* those who have early (0–6 months) post-ECT relapse not controlled by medication
* those with later recurrence (6–12 months) not controlled by medication
* those who cannot tolerate prophylactic medication
* those who repeatedly relapse because of poor compliance
* those who ask for it.

Maintenance ECT is usually reserved for those whose illness recurs after continuation ECT. Either may also be considered for patients who express a preference for them.

Assessment

Before commencing continuation ECT, a full review of the case should be undertaken in a similar manner to any case of refractory or relapsing depression. Consideration should be given to ensuring the diagnosis is correct, that ECT has been proven to be of benefit and that alternative options have been adequately explored. The patient's informed consent will need to be sought, after provision of a separate information sheet. If the patient is currently unwell, discussing continuation treatment should be deferred until he or she is sufficiently improved to allow a full understanding of the proposed plan. A specific consent form for continuation/maintenance ECT should be considered.

Once the decision to proceed has been made, the patient should have a full routine medical screening and examination, ideally performed in collaboration with an experienced anaesthetist. Electrocardiogram and chest radiography may be needed. Baseline standardised assessment of illness severity should also be performed (e.g. Hamilton Rating Scale for Depression, Montgomery–Asberg Depression Rating Scale). It would seem wise to seek a second opinion about continuation ECT from a consultant colleague, preferably one with experience in ECT. This is not a statutory requirement for an informal patient.

Exclusion criteria

Exclusion criteria for continuation ECT are the same for acute ECT – recent myocardial infarction or cerebrovascular accident, raised intracranial pressure or presence of an acute respiratory infection. One should, however, be more cautious where the use of acute ECT is of higher risk, for example with patients who have in the past shown significant post-ECT confusion or who have a depressive illness in the context of a progressive neurodegenerative disorder.

Treatment plan

Before starting continuation treatment, consideration should be given to the intended length of the course. The team should also agree on which symptoms would indicate a deterioration in the mental state such that a relapse would seem likely to occur. This information can then be used in determining the frequency of treatment. Once completed, the plan should be clearly and explicitly documented in the notes.

A full discussion with the patient and family must be conducted to address treatment purpose, benefits, adverse effects and so on, and details of this similarly documented.

ECT procedure

The administration of ECT should proceed as recommended in the Royal College of Psychiatrists' guidelines on ECT in either in-patient or out-patient setting. The goals of continuation ECT are such that out-patient treatment would be the normal pattern once recovery is achieved. Separate protocols will be needed for this locally. Electrode placement will generally be the same as used during the acute phase, although changes may be necessary.

Ideally a stimulus-dosing paradigm should be employed with the goal of inducing a seizure of between 20 to 50 seconds in length. During longer courses of ECT, seizure threshold rises, so slight increases in the dose given may be required. However, experience suggests that clinical response is a more important indicator of efficacy than seizure duration and shorter seizures can be acceptable if the patient remains well. Once the clinical recovery has occurred with ECT being given twice weekly, the goal should then be to reduce the frequency of ECT to the minimum required to maintain clinical response. This will be influenced by physical and psychological factors in each individual, so a rigid structure to treatment is inappropriate. We would suggest:

- give as acute ECT until a clinical response is achieved
- reduce to weekly
- reduce to every 10 days
- reduce to every 2 weeks
- reduce to every 3 weeks
- reduce to monthly.

Administration of treatments less frequently than monthly may be possible in certain cases. In patients who are not commencing continuation ECT immediately after acute ECT it may be possible to begin at a lower frequency, of around every 2 weeks. Routine review of efficacy should be undertaken after every two sessions in the first instance and review of frequency monthly. Once a regimen is established, review may be possible less often – as for patients on other forms of prophylaxis.

Consideration should be given to concurrent medication that may interfere with longer-term treatment. Since the ECT is being used as a prophylactic, it may be possible to reduce or withdraw psychotropics completely, although, given the severity of illness in continuation patients, a 'pure' ECT prophylaxis is often not achieved. If possible, benzodiazepines and anticonvulsants should be stopped, as they interfere with seizure activity. The majority of neuroleptics are proconvulsant. Lithium can cause significant post-ECT confusion and must be used only with caution. Non-psychiatric medications should be discussed with the anaesthetists.

Before each change in the frequency of ECT, a full review should take place. For those patients who are in an out-patient setting, objective information will be needed from community staff or family. Feedback from carers, either formal or informal, is essential. Deterioration in mental state that suggests the return of a depressive disorder at any treatment frequency should result in a return to the previous level until improvement is re-established.

Review during the course

Once initial recovery – assessed either clinically and/or by significant reduction in rating scale score – has been achieved, a full baseline psychometric assessment should be performed. This should allow assessment of current and past functioning and also be able to detect change. We would suggest testing premorbid intelligence (e.g. Weschler Adult Intelligence Scale – Revised, National Adult Reading Test), memory (e.g. Weschler Memory Scale – Revised, Rey Figure) and language (e.g. Graded Naming Test, Token Test, Verbal Fluency Test).

Routine monthly cognitive assessment (e.g. Folstein Mini-Mental State Examination) should be done as a rough guide to cognitive performance. There is a need to be aware of practice effects. At each review, information about side-effects should be sought, particularly subjective cognitive problems. For practical purposes, a senior psychiatrist can undertake routine regular review on the day of the treatment (before its administration).

There should be a full anaesthetic review by a senior anaesthetist (with laboratory tests as appropriate) every 6 months and full repeat of all psychometric assessments (excluding the National Adult Reading Test) every 12 months.

Regular review by nursing and medical staff is essential, and it is advisable to update the general practitioner at intervals. Informal verbal consent should be sought before each treatment. Written consent should be obtained at regular intervals – perhaps every 6 months or every 6 treatments.

Stopping continuation ECT

Reduction in the frequency of the ECT should continue until a stable state is reached, where there is the maximum spacing between treatments without return of symptoms. Allowing for individual variation, monthly is an appropriate goal. Since relapse is most likely within the first 12 months of recovery, it is wise to employ continuation ECT for at least 1 year after recovery, with reviews as above. At the end of this period, a full review of the need for long-term ECT should take place, that includes consultation with the patient, carers and staff involved.

If the course were begun to prevent relapse (continuation ECT), it is reasonable to consider terminating the course at this stage. With maintenance ECT, however, the use of ECT to prevent further episodes would suggest the course should be continued indefinitely. Even so, a full review at this stage must be considered advisable. Further maintenance treatment should be monitored as above.

There is currently no way of predicting how likely a relapse or recurrence is following the withdrawal of continuation ECT. Clinical predictors of relapse will be idiosyncratic to the individual patient. Hence the need for careful documenting of each patient's particular symptoms initially. We would suggest that close clinical supervision is maintained in the period after a course and that return of symptoms would indicate consideration of maintenance ECT. Once this decision is made, regular review should continue as above, with annual review of its role.

Legal issues

If acute ECT given under the Mental Health Act is effective, it should be possible to establish informal status and informed consent before or early in the continuation phase. If this cannot be done, it is unlikely that the treatment is working and its use should be reassessed.

While there is no theoretical reason why continuation ECT cannot be given under Mental Health Act following a second opinion, this situation should be viewed with caution. If the patient does not respond sufficiently to develop capacity to consent, then the role of ECT is not clear. Also, giving ECT as a prophylactic to a recovered patient without informed consent has questionable legality. It has recently been suggested that it is legal (in England and Wales) to administer ECT to an incapacitated compliant patient in the absence of consent without recourse to the Mental Health Act under the doctrine of clinical necessity (Jones, 1999). Although arguably legal, practitioners may feel uncomfortable with this position. Extending this argument, it might be suggested that continuation ECT could be given to prevent deterioration in the condition of an incapacitated compliant patient with only inferred consent. Such a situation might arise in a demented depressed patient whose clinical condition is clearly much improved after ECT but who rapidly deteriorates without it. There seems to be no case law covering this situation.

As already mentioned, a separate consent form for patients consenting to a course of continuation ECT is advised. The consent needs to be reaffirmed every 6 months or after a fixed number of treatments (probably 6).

Reference

Jones, R. (1999) *The Mental Health Act Manual* (6th edn), pp. 240–241. London: Sweet and Maxwell.

Richard Barnes
January 2005

Suppliers of ECT machines in the UK

Dantec Dynamics Ltd
Garonor Way
Royal Portbury
Bristol
BS20 7XE

Tel: 01275 375 333
Fax: 01275 375 336

web: www.dantecdynamics.co.uk

Ectron Ltd
Knap Close
Letchworth
Herts
SG6 1AQ

Tel: 01462 682 124
Fax: 01462 481 463

Oxford Instruments Medical Ltd
Manor Way
Old Woking
Surrey
GU22 9JU

Tel: 01483 770 331
Fax: 01483 727 193

Email: sales.msd@oxinst.co.uk
Web: www.oxinst.com

Inspection of ECT clinics

In May 2003 the Royal College of Psychiatrists launched a new ECT Accreditation Service (ECTAS) to coincide with the publication of the NICE guidance. The aim was to raise standards in the administration of ECT and the new service was to be managed by the College Research Unit. Further background information is available on the College website (www.rcpsych.ac.uk/press/preleases/pr/pr_413.htm). Details of the accreditation process and the latest ECTAS standards are available from the College website (www.rcpsych.ac.uk/cru/ECTAS.htm).

ECTAS does not extend to Scotland, where the Scottish ECT Audit Network (SEAN) continues to operate. The network has its own website (www.sean.org.uk) and the SEAN standards and audit materials are also available to download (www.sean.org.uk/amats.php).

Index

Compiled by Caroline Sheard